i

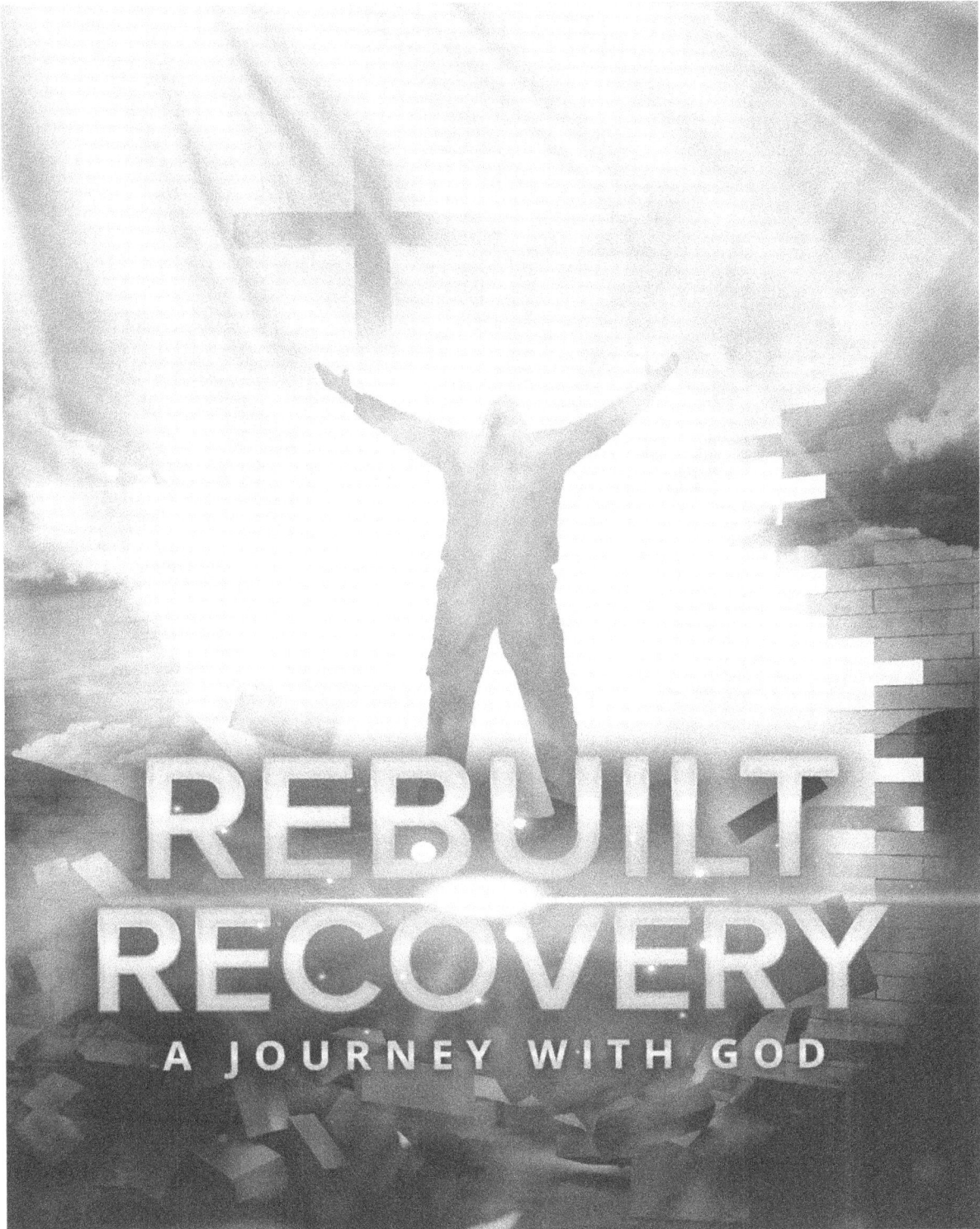

REBUILT
RECOVERY
A JOURNEY WITH GOD

Glorious Hope Publishing

New Carlisle, Ohio

# Rebuilt Recovery

## A Journey with God

## Book 4 – Your Journey Home

By: Heather L. Phipps

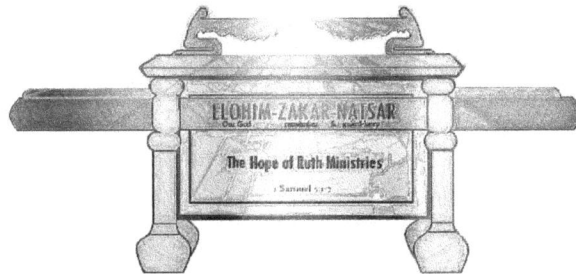

Rebuilt Recovery Is a Ministry of The Hope of Ruth Ministries Church

Glorious Hope Publishing

Glorious Hope Publishing
Hope of Ruth Ministries
307 Prentice Dr. New Carlisle, Ohio 45344
info@hopeofruthministries.com
www.hopeofruthministries.com

*Thank you to the following people
who gave their ideas, hearts,
and lives into making this book possible.*

Cindy Varghese

Summer Curtis

Alysha Allen

Justin Curtis

Annaka Schleinitz-Brooks

Jaycie Curtis

Camie Hawkins

Terri Allison

# Contents

# The Complete Rebuilt Series

## Boxes and Symbols

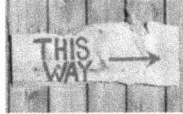

These boxes have thoughts or questions involving your coach.

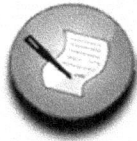

These boxes contain additional tasks for your journey.
Do not skip these tasks!

These boxes contain tips with additional information to help understand or implement the topic being discussed.

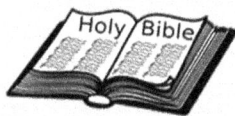

This icon indicates scripture important to understanding the current topic.

These boxes have important points for you to consider.

"These boxes contain interesting quotes"

# Disclaimer

The information contained in the *Rebuilt for Life* (online course), *Rebuilt Recovery*, or *Rebuilt Website* is for general information purposes only. The content is not intended to be a substitute for professional advice, diagnosis, or treatment, rather it is intended as a supplement to it. Always seek the advice of your mental health professional or other qualified health provider with any questions you may have regarding your condition. It is your responsibility to inform your mental health professional that you are using a *Rebuilt* service to aid your recovery. Never disregard professional advice or delay in seeking it because of something you have read or heard in *Rebuilt* materials, website, or courses.

> If you are in crisis or have an emergency, call 911 immediately.
>
> **If you have suicidal thoughts, call the National Suicide Prevention Lifeline 1-800-273-TALK (8255) to talk with a skilled, trained counselor at a crisis center in your area.**
>
> **If you are located outside the United States, call your local emergency line immediately.**

**Rebuilt coaches are not qualified counselors and do not take the place of certified professionals.**

The information is provided by *The Hope of Ruth Ministries* and whilst we endeavor to keep the information up-to-date and correct, we make no representations or warranties of any kind, express or implied, about the completeness, accuracy, reliability, suitability, or availability with respect to the website, books, online course, the information, products, services, or related graphics contained on the internet or print materials for any purpose. Any reliance you place on such information is therefore strictly at your own risk.

In no event will we be liable for any loss or damage including without limitation, indirect or consequential injury, loss, or damage, or any injury, loss, or damage whatsoever arising from loss of life, relations, property, data, or profits arising out of, or in connection with, the use of the *Rebuilt* website, *Rebuilt for Life*, *Rebuilt Recovery*, or *Rebuilt Coaches*.

Every effort is made to keep the websites up and running smoothly. However, *The Hope of Ruth Ministries* nor *Rebuilt Recovery* takes no responsibility for, and will not be liable for, the coaches, website, software, or course being temporarily unavailable due to technical issues beyond our control.

## COPYRIGHT NOTICE FOR SUPPLEMENTAL MATERIAL

## EXTERNAL LINKS

Through the *Rebuilt* websites and courses, you may link to other websites, which are not under the control of *Rebuilt* or *The Hope of Ruth Ministries*.  We have no control over the nature, content, and availability of such sites.  The inclusion of any links does not necessarily imply a recommendation or endorse the views expressed within them.

# Serenity Prayer

God, grant me the serenity
to accept the things I cannot change,
the courage to change the things I can,
and the wisdom to know the difference.

Living one day at a time,
enjoying one moment at a time;
accepting hardship as a pathway
to peace;

taking, as Jesus did,
this sinful world as it is,
not as I would have it;
trusting that You will make
all things right
if I surrender to Your will;

so that I may be reasonably happy
in this life
and supremely happy with You
forever in the next.

Amen.

**Reinhold Niebuhr**

# Introduction to Book Four

## Your Journey Home — The Future

You have learned many things through this journey: how to love yourself, identify the enemy's lies, trust God in your hurt, and turn to Him when you mess up. You walk through life with the Lord by your side. Remember how far you have come!

As you begin this book, you might be experiencing a mixture of emotions. You may feel confident in your progress and ready for this journey to end, or you may be concerned about repeating past mistakes and questioning your ability to discern truth from lies. This book will help you hone the skills needed to maintain your victory, stay confident, and prevent a relapse into old thinking.

The enemy is always in your ear, wanting you to fail, but you know a secret: He loses! God turns his plans upside down. All the enemy meant for your destruction becomes your blessing. You will not fear falling when you remain diligent and keep your eyes on your source.

The close of one journey begins another. Your relationship with the Lord grows deeper as your life begins to flow forth from His. The lessons in this book will teach you to fight spiritual enemies, have strong relationships, handle conflict, and step forward.

## In This Book

**Your Journey Home**
You have a hidden enemy trying to sabotage your future. Conquer your flesh by making the Lord your only stronghold.

**Choosing Healthy Relationships**
Learn about healthy and toxic relationships, and about setting boundaries. You will also learn how to identify detrimental behaviors in yourself and others.

**Conflict Resolution**
An in-depth look at resolving conflicts and establishing effective communication.

**Moving Forward**
Learn to live *from* God instead of *for* Him. Establish useful habits to protect your focus from slipping. Write your story and discover ways to serve with *Rebuilt*.

# Chapter Sixteen

# Your Journey Home

# Lesson 41 — Your Journey Home

How do you feel knowing your time with *Rebuilt* is coming to an end? It is the close of one season in a lifelong quest. Your growth does not cease when you complete the last page of this book. The deep-rooted sin and strongholds interwoven in your heart are difficult to pull out. You may notice you are continuing to be tested in old strongholds and problematic thinking patterns, or you may discover new ones. This is the Lord's way to **fortify your freedom** and **strengthen your faith** in Him. The tools you have learned have set you on the right course to weather future challenges and make the Lord your only stronghold.

*The Lord is my light and my salvation; whom shall I fear?*
*The Lord is the stronghold of my life; of whom shall I be afraid? (Psalm 27:1)*

*The Lord is a stronghold for the oppressed a stronghold in times of trouble. And those*
*who know your name put their trust in you, for you, O Lord, have not forsaken those who*
*seek you. (Psalm 9:9 – 10)*

## Process of Progress

Healing the hurts in your heart is like cleaning out a physical wound. Slapping a bandage over a serious wound without giving it proper care and treatment traps all the yuck inside, allowing infection to fester and spread to the rest of the body. To properly care for a wound, you must cleanse it thoroughly. You must debride the wound to prevent any infection from remaining. The deeper the wound, the deeper you must go to clear it out.

In the past you used many things, perhaps even Jesus, as a Band-Aid® to cover emotional and spiritual wounds without dealing with the root or cause of the injury. Just as with physical injuries, the longer you allow an emotional hurt to fester, the more digging is required to remove the corruption it caused.

By this point, you have **pulled off your emotional bandage, cut away the damage, and cleared the festering infection underneath.** You no longer cover up your wounds, pretend they do not exist, or believe they can improve on their own. But even with proper treatment, deep emotional trauma takes time to heal. You may experience complete freedom in some areas while infection is still being purged in others. The process peels back layer after layer until the Lord reveals every hidden poison in your heart.

**This book will serve as an aid to strengthen and prepare you for the continuing journey ahead.** The principles presented here are meant to help you **prevent relapse** and **continue the healing process.** You will further your relationship with God, develop healthy relationships, establish reasonable boundaries, and foster better communication.

## Where Are You?

You made considerable progress on this journey. Before continuing, take a moment to assess your growth. This will prepare you to deal with future struggles and give you confidence in your successes. **For each question that follows, state how much you thought or believed the idea before you started this journey, and how much you believe the idea now. Is there a large change? Are there areas where you would like to see more change?**

<u>Questions to Ponder</u>

Provide two answers for each question below, one for before you started this journey and one for where you are now. State your answers as either percentages, or on a scale of 1 to 10, with 1 being not at all and 10 being the maximum amount.

41.1) How well did/do you learn from your failures?

41.2) How often did/are you choosing change (doing and thinking differently)?

41.3) How much were/are you living for God?

41.4) How much were/are you living to survive?

41.5) How much did/do you trust God's Word is true *for you*?

41.6) How secure were/are you in your relationship with God?

41.7) How much trust did/do you give God?

41.8) How often did/do you hear God's voice?

41.9) Were/Are you bandaging your wounds or facing them?

41.10) How much did/do you believe that God invests in you? Explain.

Consider your responses to the previous questions when answering the following.

41.11) In what ways do you trust God, both now and before your journey began?

41.12) In what areas do you recognize the most change since beginning *Rebuilt*?

41.13) In which areas do you note the most change?

41.14) In which areas do you note the least change?

41.15) Where would you prefer to see more change or improvement?

## Where Are You Headed?

Head for the finish line! This life is a race to eternity, a training ground for our future. The prize? A crown, a kingdom, an eternal existence with no pain or tears. Keep your eyes on the prize. God's Word says not to grow weary of doing good. Do not give up! Stand firm and confident!

*Do you not know that in a race all the runners run, but only one receives the prize? So run that you may obtain it. Every athlete exercises self-control in all things. They do it to receive a perishable wreath, but we imperishable. (1 Corinthians 9:24 – 25)*

*I have fought the good fight, I have finished the race, I have kept the faith. (2 Timothy 4:7)*

*And I am sure of this, that he who began a good work in you will bring it to completion at the day of Jesus Christ. (Philippians 1:6)*

*And let us not grow weary of doing good, for in due season we will reap, if we do not give up. (Galatians 6:9)*

<u>Questions to Ponder</u>

41.16) How have your priorities changed? Define your priorities for the future.

41.17) How do you see your life unfolding differently after *Rebuilt*?

41.18) How does this differ from what you expected for your life before you began *Rebuilt*?

# Lesson 42 — A Surprising Enemy

You have a spiritual enemy who hates you, especially because of your relationship with the Lord. He will do anything to make you ineffective in God's Kingdom. To combat this enemy, you must first understand him. **His main stomping ground is the undisciplined mind.** He speaks lies and tempts us, **but it is our choices, not Satan, that make us sin.**

Your thoughts and desires birth sin. Satan inhabits your sin, using it as a doorway into your life. Satan capitalizes on your fearful or wrong thinking to conceive desires, tempting you to act on sinful thoughts (i.e., any thought which goes against the Word of God). He uses the sin in you to steal, kill, and destroy.

> *But each person is tempted when he is <u>lured and enticed by his own desire</u>. Then desire when it has conceived gives birth to sin, and sin when it is fully grown brings forth death.*
> *(James 1:14 – 15)*

**Sin** is the **power** behind your **enemy,** but **we have free will.** When we **choose life and live**, the Lord will take what Satan meant to destroy us and use it for our good.

> *I call heaven and earth to witness against you today, that I have set before you life and death, blessing and curse. Therefore choose life, that you and your offspring may live.*
> *(Deuteronomy 30:19)*

God's word tells us to have the mind of Christ because the mind is where our battle begins. Satan whispers lies in our ear, but with the mind of Christ, sin is dead in us and Satan's influence diminishes. When we have the Lord, we recognize that our greatest enemy is our own flesh.

> *Since therefore Christ suffered in the flesh, <u>arm yourselves with the same way of thinking</u>, for whoever has <u>suffered in the flesh has ceased from sin</u>, so as to live for the rest of the time in the flesh no longer for human passions but for the will of God. (1 Peter 4:1 – 2)*

Having the mind of Christ is not considering ourselves equal with God; rather, it is exalting God and emptying ourselves to be filled with His Spirit. We exchange our own ways, thoughts, and desires for God's ways, thoughts, and desires.

> *<u>Have this mind among yourselves, which is\ yours in Christ Jesus</u>, who, though he was in the form of God, did not count equality with God a thing to be grasped, but emptied himself, by taking the form of a servant, being born in the likeness of men. (Philippians 2:5 – 7)*

Jesus served as our example. He emptied himself, sacrificing his divine position to be born a man, and he was humbled, even to death on a cross. He subjected any desire of His flesh in obedience to the Father's will, and God exalted him for this. Jesus knew **humanity's greatest struggle** was trying to grasp equality with God—a goal we could never attain. Since the enemy tempted Eve with the words "you will be like God, knowing good and evil" (Genesis 3:5), we all fight against this same sin. We want to be **God over our own self, our own purpose, and our own thoughts**. When you realize you will never be God and empty yourself, **God will exalt you**.

Having a mind like Christ means our ways are acceptable to our righteous God. If Jesus were sitting next to you, would you watch that movie with Him? Would you listen to that music or play that game? Would you speak the way you speak to others? What about the thoughts in your mind? Would you speak those thoughts out loud to Jesus? Is your anger righteous?

A disciplined mind is crucial to your continuing walk with the Lord!

### Questions to Ponder

42.1) **Consider your recent actions, thoughts, and words. Write both positive and negative examples of each.**

42.2) **In what situations were you negative?**

42.3) **When do the opinions of men guide you instead of the opinions of God?**

Examine your answers above. For each item you mentioned:

42.4) **In what ways did you have a mind like Christ?**

42.5) **In what ways are you trying to be God over your own life or other situations?**

## Patience Please, Your Flesh Is Fighting for Survival

*For I do not understand my own actions. For I do not do what I want, but I do the very thing I hate. Now if I do what I do not want, I agree with the law, that it is good. So now it is no longer I who do it, but sin that dwells within me. For I know that nothing good dwells in me, that is, in my flesh. For I have the desire to do what is right, but not the ability to carry it out. For I do not do the good I want, but the evil I do not want is what I keep on doing. Now if I do what I do not want, it is no longer I who do it, but sin that dwells within me. (Romans 7:15 – 20)*

Freedom comes as the Lord removes the root of the wrong thoughts that cause our sin. When we suffer in the flesh and overcome, **we cease sinning** in that area. The power of sin still works in areas of our life in which we continue acting in wrong, harmful ways. Have patience with your suffering flesh; it is dying to sin, and it wants to live. Remember, when your heart's desire is to do right, but you still do wrong, **your mistakes do not define you**. It is your sin nature.

## The True Replacement Theology

The blood of Jesus makes us righteous. He paid the price to remove our sin from us. Why does it matter when we continue to sin if He forgives it?

*If we say we have no sin, we deceive ourselves, and the truth is not in us. (1 John 1:8)*

As Christians, we are being transformed into a bride without blemish, suitable to marry a king! We were **made righteous** by Jesus' sacrifice, and we are **being made holy**, set apart for the Lord. By following Christ, our lives reflect a transformation that serves as a witness of Him to the world. God promises to continue **taking us from one measure of glory to the next**.

*And we all, with unveiled face, beholding the glory of the Lord, are being transformed into the same image from one degree of glory to another. For this comes from the Lord who is the Spirit. (2 Corinthians 3:18)*

*And I am sure of this, that he who began a good work in you will bring it to completion at the day of Jesus Christ. (Philippians 1:6)*

## The Replacement

If we are to become the new creation in Christ, **God must replace our sin nature with His nature** by a process of put-offs and put-ons, replacing our old ways with new. **Both natures cannot exist together.** Scripture shows this process through a vision of Joshua, the high priest.

> *Then he showed me Joshua the high priest standing before the angel of the LORD, and Satan standing at his right hand to accuse him. And the LORD said to Satan, "The LORD rebuke you, O Satan! The LORD who has chosen Jerusalem rebuke you! Is not this a brand plucked from the fire?" Now Joshua was standing before the angel, clothed with filthy garments. And the angel said to those who were standing before him, "Remove the filthy garments from him." And to him he said, "Behold, I have taken your iniquity away from you, and I will clothe you with pure vestments." And I said, "Let them put a clean turban on his head." So they put a clean turban on his head and clothed him with garments. And the angel of the LORD was standing by. (Zechariah 3:1 – 5)*

This passage paints a symbolic picture of our transformation into a "new man." Satan and the Lord are arguing for Joshua. The Lord removes his filthy garments (the sin nature), replacing them with pure vestments (righteousness). **It is not enough to stop sinning. We must replace what we cast off with something new: Christ.**

In the New Testament, Paul teaches us what things we should put off or put on using the Greek word *enduo*. It refers to putting on and taking off clothing. Paul is addressing both what must be removed from our lives, like filthy garments, and in what we should clothe ourselves.

Consider your routine when you get up in the morning to start your day as a picture of God's plan for redemption. First, you take off your dirty clothes. This is like when you realize you must turn away from your sin. Then you hop in the shower. This is like when begin to become spiritually clean by acknowledging the sacrifice of Jesus to pay the price of your sin. You are clean, but before you are free to go, you must get dressed.

After you bathe, you put on undergarments so your clothing fits properly. This is like putting on Christ and abiding in Him. **Righteousness will not fit well unless Jesus is your foundation.** Now you are ready to get dressed in righteousness to head outside. In a spiritual sense, this is the armor of God, the outer covering that protects you from the tactics of your enemy and accuser.

---

*There are many spiritual outfits we can wear as believers: garments of praise, garments of salvation, wedding garments, robes of dedication, the covering of a cloak, and so on. Throughout Scripture, there are references to wearing, changing, putting on, or taking off different garments. These can represent many things, but they generally apply to an aspect of our character or actions and relate back to our relationship with God. Garments in Scripture may have a negative connotation, such as filthy garments. You can learn a lot from an in-depth study on this topic, but for now, our focus will be on those things that we are instructed to put on or put off in the New Testament.*

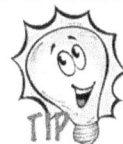

## The Wardrobe

**When you dress well, people take notice.** The same is true when it comes to your spiritual "clothing." Your armor becomes a witness of Christ to the world. Your completed wardrobe prepares you to experience the abundant life God promises. Fully dressed, you live in peace, allow your faith to grow, cling to the Word, hold firm to your salvation, love the truth, and pursue righteousness. Now you are ready to be God's ambassador, representing Him in freedom.

## Your Wardrobe with Christ

➢ Put off your old self (your flesh) and put on your new self (the likeness of Christ).

*Do not lie to one another, seeing that you have put off the old self with its practices and have put on the new self, which is being renewed in knowledge after the image of its creator. (Colossians 3:9 – 10)*

*To put off your old self, which belongs to your former manner of life and is corrupt through deceitful desires, and to be renewed in the spirit of your minds, and to put on the new self, created after the likeness of God in true righteousness and holiness. (Ephesians 4:22 – 24)*

➢ Dress yourself in Christ each day.

*For as many of you as were baptized into Christ have put on Christ. (Galatians 3:27)*

*But put on the Lord Jesus Christ, and make no provision for the flesh, to gratify its desires. (Romans 13:14)*

➢ Put off sin and the passions, temptations, and old practices of the flesh.

*Therefore put away all filthiness and rampant wickedness and receive with meekness the implanted word, which is able to save your souls. (James 1:21)*

*So put away all malice and all deceit and hypocrisy and envy and all slander. (1 Peter 2:1)*

*Therefore, having put away falsehood, let each one of you speak the truth with his neighbor, for we are members one of another. (Ephesians 4:25)*

*The night is far gone; the day is at hand. So then let us cast off the works of darkness and put on the armor of light. (Romans 13:12)*

➢ Put **on** love, light, the new self, godly character, and virtues.

*Put on then, as God's chosen ones, holy and beloved, compassionate hearts, kindness, humility, meekness, and patience. (Colossians 3:12)*

*And above all these put on love, which binds everything together in perfect harmony. (Colossians 3:14)*

*For in this tent we groan, longing to put on our heavenly dwelling, if indeed by putting it on we may not be found naked. For while we are still in this tent, we groan, being burdened—not that we would be unclothed, but that we would be further clothed, so that what is mortal may be swallowed up by life. For in this tent we groan, longing to put on our heavenly dwelling. (2 Corinthians 5:2)*

> Put on your full set of armor so you can stand firm and not give the enemy a place.

> *Therefore take up the whole armor of God, that you may be able to withstand in the evil day, and having done all, to stand firm. Stand therefore, having fastened on the belt of truth, and having put on the breastplate of righteousness, and, as shoes for your feet, having put on the readiness given by the gospel of peace. In all circumstances take up the shield of faith, with which you can extinguish all the flaming darts of the evil one; and take the helmet of salvation, and the sword of the Spirit, which is the word of God, praying at all times in the Spirit, with all prayer and supplication. (Ephesians 6:13 – 18)*

It is often difficult to do right; the battle with our flesh is real. Paul told us in 1 Corinthians 9:27, *"But I discipline my body and keep it under control, lest after preaching to others I myself should be disqualified."* The word Paul used for discipline implies he is beating his flesh black and blue to keep it under control so as not to damage his witness for Christ.

> *And let us not grow weary of doing good, for in due season we will reap, if we do not give up. (Galatians 6:9)*

## Questions to Ponder

42.6) Do you have a constant back-and-forth struggle between living for Christ and living for your flesh? Describe your own struggle with your flesh.

42.7) What thoughts or feelings may cause you to give place to the enemy?

42.8) Is there something you hold as an idol above God? (This could be a person, desire, ideal, thought, emotion, or stronghold.)

42.9) Is there sin in your life that you keep returning to? What do you need to "put off"?

42.10) Considering your progress, what do you still need to "put on" to replace old hang-ups?

---

In your Journal, record potential future stumbling-blocks that you may have discovered in this lesson.

What spiritual clothing will you dress in to replace old beliefs and habits?

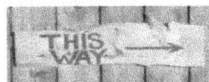

---

### Your coach has an activity for you this week.

When Christ died for our sins, he took everything of our old self. It was not just sins nailed to that cross, but the result of our sin nature. Your shame, pride, anger, insecurity, anxiety, pain, depression, and labels no longer belong to you. They died on the cross with Jesus. His death made all things new. One day, we will fully transform into Christ's likeness, and there will be no trace of our sin nature left.

**Look for sins, pride, control, negativity. Listen for times when you say or think, "I am _____." Each time you are rejecting who you are, remember the I AM placed your "bad" on His shoulders to be crucified with Him.**

# Chapter Seventeen

## Choosing Healthy Relationships

# A Very Important Chapter!

## Why Focus on Relationships?

**Relationship is the key to recovery.** Relationship with God foremost, then relationship with self, and now relationships with others. Think back on your journey. You are likely to discover most of your trouble and pain originated **directly or indirectly** with other people. It is vital to build healthy relationships, identify toxic behaviors, communicate well, and handle conflict biblically **to prevent falling away from God and relapse**.

Healthy, caring relationships add a rich blessing to your life. Challenging times are not so difficult when you have someone by your side. Yet the most tender, loving relationships can cause you the most pain when you feel betrayed, rejected, or left behind by your loved one(s). Unavoidable pain is part of this life. Jesus understands these hurts, as He too experienced rejection, betrayal, and loss. **He helps you through these situations.** You are not alone.

Relationships can be toxic or dysfunctional. God's Word gives you all the aid you need to avoid or navigate these types of relationships. **The people with whom you associate matter to God and to your recovery.** People have a significant influence in your life and may lead you to question your value and worth. Toxic people dump their burdens on your shoulders, judge you, lie to you, reject you, harm you, and use and manipulate you. The effects of another's sin have a far reach, often right into your heart.

Through this journey, you have learned how important it is to love yourself. You understand that your worth and value are inherent to you, not dependent on your success or another's opinions of your worth. This alone is a powerful aid to building healthy relationships. One of Satan's greatest tools is your fear of rejection and shame. **Without that influence, the fear of man loses its power**, and God's voice becomes clear. Healthy boundaries help you identify and cut loose from the bondage of toxic relationships. Effective communication makes misunderstandings less likely to cause pain and division.

People's words and actions affect our lives. The way you deal with life issues either makes you victorious or destroys you. Handling conflict God's way will insulate you from the negative effects of people-problems while developing a Christ-like character in you and keeping you safe. **Engaging in healthy conflict is a way to show love to yourself.** The objective of recovery is **not to avoid pain and conflict.** Rather, the goal is to walk through your trials confident in God's protection.

You can have confidence in God's help. Recall Jesus' prayer for His believers in John 17:

*I have given them your word, and the world has hated them because they are not of the world, just as I am not of the world. I do not ask that you take them out of the world, but that you keep them from the evil one. (John 17:14 – 15)*

13

# Lesson 43 — Circles of Relationship

Nothing feels more rewarding than a healthy relationship, or more devastating than an unhealthy one. Are you pursuing a friendship with someone who should be an acquaintance? We long for close, real companionship, for another person to fully know us, but Jesus should fill those needs first. Moving forward with Christ may mean reevaluating your relationships.

Relationship is the giving of your heart to another. Therefore, this lesson defines relationship by how much you <u>trust another with your heart</u> and <u>not by marital or blood relation</u>.

## What Is a Friend?

In our culture, we often call anyone we know a friend. Friends may be related to you, but not all your relatives are your friends. Scripture warns us about having too many people we call friends. You may have 500 or 1,000 friends on social media, but are they authentic friendships? Most people we call friend we should really consider acquaintances.

*A man of many companions may come to ruin, but there is a friend who sticks closer than a brother. (Proverbs 18:24)*

Throughout Scripture, examples of friendship share one commonality: They are all sacrificial relationships. True friends are rare. You may have only one person in your life that you could consider a genuine friend. A friend lays down his or her right to retribution, to be self-seeking, and hide behind walls. A friend knows your innermost you. They show loyalty, devotion, and dependability. A friend gives wise counsel that leads you to the Lord and righteousness. They will *not* always agree with you, and they do not smother you in flattery. These are the people you want in your inner circle.

This level of friendship bears lasting fruit. Examples in Scripture show that friendship is the greatest connection, the greatest love you can have for another person. Friendship is reciprocal and sacrificial. One beautiful illustration of friendship in Scripture is that of Jonathan and David. The Lord knit their souls together. What hurt one hurt the other. What rejoiced one gave joy to the other. They would sacrifice for one another, even to their own detriment.

*As soon as he had finished speaking to Saul, the soul of Jonathan was knit to the soul of David, and Jonathan loved him as his own soul. (1Samuel 18:1)*

Scripture shows us another such friendship in the relationship between Naomi and her daughter-in-law, Ruth. After the death of their husbands, Naomi directed Ruth to return to her people to protect her from a life of hardship. Ruth refused to go, showing loyalty to Naomi, and illustrating a friendship forged in the love of God.

*But Ruth said, "Do not urge me to leave you or to return from following you. For where you go I will go, and where you lodge I will lodge. Your people shall be my people, and your God my God. Where you die I will die, and there will I be buried. May the LORD do so to me and more also if anything but death parts me from you. (Ruth 1:16 – 17)*

The reward of genuine friendship is two lives knitted together and love greater than any other relationship, apart from the love of Jesus. Friendship is not just about what one does for or gives to the other. **Friends reciprocate with selfless love, joy, trust, belonging, companionship, and loyalty, sharing their lives, and being known by one another.**

## What Is an Acquaintance?

Most of your relationships may not fit this definition of friendship. Instead, they are probably acquaintances. These are folks you interact with on a regular basis but **cannot trust with the innermost parts of your heart**. An acquaintance may be a relative, or someone with whom you minister, work, or socialize, but **lack a reciprocal or sacrificial relationship**.

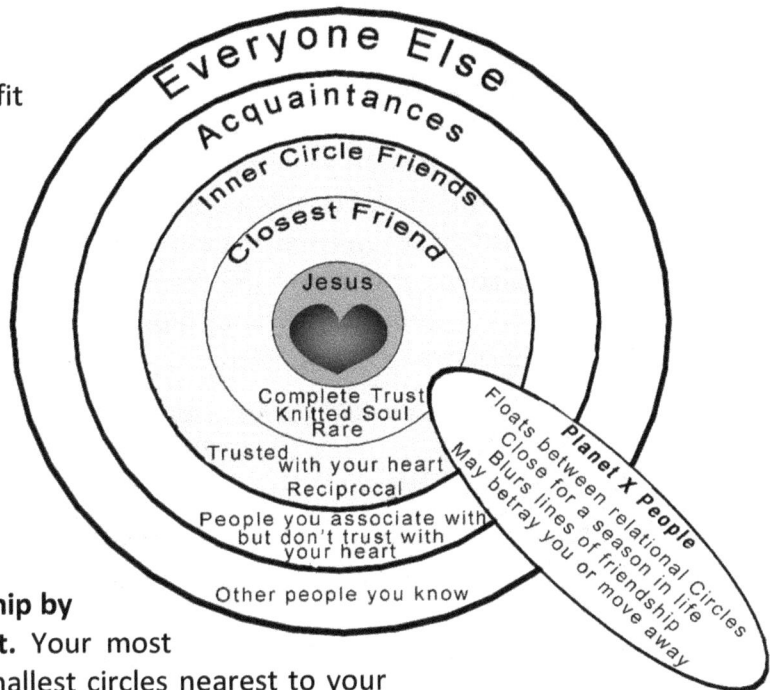

## The Q Chart

**The Q chart shows circles of relationship by how close a person is to your heart.** Your most trusted and closest people are the smallest circles nearest to your heart. **The nearer a person is to your heart, the more vulnerable you become.** Yet these are the most rewarding relationships. Notice that **the closer it gets to your heart, the smaller the circle is.** Larger circles represent more people than the smaller circles.

**Here is what these circles represent:**

- The shaded area represents your inner circle.

- The center circle represents your heart, and **the only one** who fits in the circle with your heart **is Jesus**. He has full access to your heart and is your first and closest friend.

- The closest friend circle has the **one** closest friend that you **absolutely trust** with your heart. This **may or may not** be a spouse or family member. This relationship represents mutual "best friendness." Having multiple people in this circle is difficult, and in most cases impossible, to maintain.

- Your next circle is your inner circle friendships. It contains certain friends or family members you **trust with your heart** but are not as close to as the person in the previous ring. They must be trustworthy, people you feel safe to confide in, and who share the same level of trust in you. **Relatives in this circle must also meet this criterion.**

- Then you have acquaintances. These are friends and relatives you spend time with for a variety of reasons. You may enjoy their company very much, but you do not give them **the same level of trust** as your inner circle friendships, **or the trust does not extend both ways**.

- The last circle contains **everyone else** you know, but with whom you lack any significant interactions.

- Then there are what we call the "Planet X People" because they break orbit. They float in and out of the different circles. **These relationships are short-term.** These folks impact your life for a season or for specific reasons. They may move away, grow distant, travel a different path in life, lack the loyalty to stick around. They may even use or betray you.

- Strangers are outside of the circle.

## Not Everyone Should Be a Friend

Genuine friendship requires **vulnerability**, and that is frightening for many people. People who have been hurt, rejected, used, or manipulated fear openness with others. Yet we rob ourselves of one of the greatest gifts God gives when we live with our hearts guarded.

**The Lord knows the risk** of opening our hearts and lives to another person, which is why **He warns us to use wisdom when choosing our friends** and warns against allowing the influence of dishonest, manipulative, or negative people into our inner circles. Friendship is always mutual. No one should coerce you into a friendship. Likewise, if your investment in someone is not reciprocated, reconsider the relationship.

> *One who is righteous is a guide to his neighbor, but the way of the wicked leads them astray.*
> *(Proverbs. 12:26)*

## Healthy Friendships

**Look at what defines a healthy friendship. Are your relationships healthy?**

- **Mutual Choice** – Friendship is not one-sided, chosen for you, or coerced through guilt or intimidation.
  *"Two are better than one, because they have a good reward for their toil"* (Ecclesiastes 4:9)

- **Mutual Benefit** – A friendship is reciprocal, not codependent. In a reciprocal relationship, both people benefit from mutual acts of love and companionship. Codependent relationships give a perceived benefit based on need or fear instead of from an overflow of genuine love.
  *"Bear one another's burdens, and so fulfill the law of Christ"* (Galatians 6:2).

- **Mutual Respect** – In a healthy friendship, each person respects the other's individuality. They accept on another's differences and decisions. They are not jealous, controlling, or judgmental, but are quick to overlook faults, give grace, and forgive generously.
  *"Do nothing from selfish ambition or conceit, but in humility count others more significant than yourselves"* (Philippians 2:3).
  *"Love one another with brotherly affection. Outdo one another in showing honor"* (Romans 12:10).

- **Mutual Concern** – Friends know each other intimately and will share their lives with one another. They hurt for one another's hurts and rejoice over one another's victories.
  *"Let each of you look not only to his own interests, but also to the interests of others"* (Philippians 2:4).

- **Mutual Beliefs** – Friends must share the same beliefs. You cannot walk through life with someone who is taking a different road.
  *"Complete my joy by being of the same mind, having the same love, being in full accord and of one mind"* (Philippians 2:2).
  *"What accord has Christ with Belial? Or what portion does a believer share with an unbeliever?"* (2 Corinthians 6:15).

- **Mutual Growth** – Friends grow together and make one another better. If you are the smartest person you know, it is time to acquire different friends.
  *"Iron sharpens iron, and one man sharpens another"* (Proverbs 27:17).
  *"And let us consider how to stir up one another to love and good works"* (Hebrews 10:24).

- **Mutual Trust** – Friends are open and truthful when they make mistakes, offend someone, or make poor choices. They put your wellbeing above their risk of rejection.
  *"Faithful are the wounds of a friend, but the kisses of an enemy are deceitful"* (Proverbs 27:6).

## Examine the relationships in your life and the way you relate to others.

Answer the questions below, then fill out your own Q chart.

### Questions to Ponder

Answer the questions below using this lesson's definitions of *friend* and *acquaintance*.

43.1) Describe the type of friend you are. How is the love of Christ evident in your friendships? Where is it missing in your friendships?

43.2) Are you the type of person you would want in your own inner circle? Why or why not?

43.3) How open are your friendships? Are your closest friendships superficial, or do you both see one another's inner man—the deepest part of who you are?

List everyone you interact with in person or on the internet. Include all relatives. Use this list to answer the questions below and fill in the Q chart.

43.4) Examine your close friendships. What level of trust do you have for each person?

43.5) It is easy to see close relatives (spouse, children, parents, siblings) through a filter of your experiences with them, yet people change and grow. Examine these relationships. What level of trust do you give each person now?

43.6) Are family members in your inner circle only because they are family? Would they hold the same role in your life if they were not related? Why or why not?

43.7) Do you have people in your life who will keep you accountable and sharpen your faith (iron sharpening iron)?

43.8) What people in your life share your beliefs and theology?

43.9) Do you have a genuine friend?

43.10) What person (or people) in your life do you need to invest in more?

43.11) Whose influence in your life sways you away from the Lord or his commands?

43.12) Are there people to whom you should minister but keep out of your inner circle?

43.13) Which relationships should you reevaluate in your life?

43.14) Is there anyone in your life with whom you should not keep close company? Is there anyone you should avoid altogether?

43.15) Would those whom you consider in your inner circle say you are in their inner circle as well?

43.16) If those in your inner circle understood how this lesson defines friendship, would they say you fit that definition of a friend in their lives? Explain the ways you fit and do not fit that definition with each person.

43.17) Jesus is in your innermost circle. Would <u>He</u> say you reciprocate that level of friendship with Him?

# Q Chart Worksheet

**Fill in the Q chart. Add names of people in your life to the proper circle.**
**Who is in your inner circle?** *(You may make copies of this page.)*

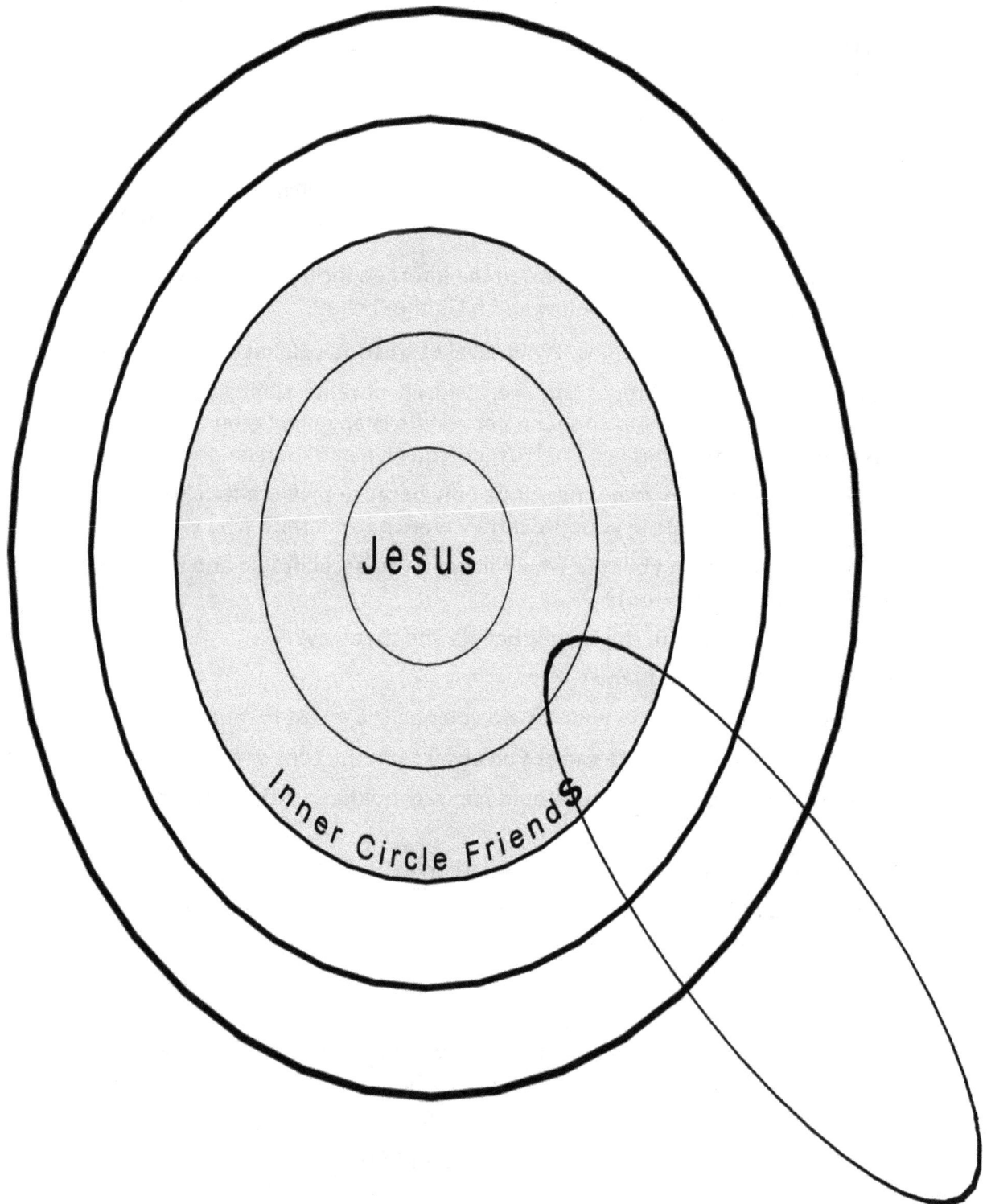

Jesus

Inner Circle Friends

# Lesson 44 — Toxic Relationships & Behaviors

People may bless your life or be a detriment. Their opinions hold much less weight when you are confident in who you are. Even so, their toxic behaviors may harm you or lead you away from doing what is right with God. Scripture tells us to avoid such people.

***As for a person who stirs up division, after warning him once and then twice, have nothing more to do with him, knowing that such a person is warped and sinful; he is self-condemned. (Titus 3:10 – 11)***

Scripture defines many types of division. These can include harsh words and manipulation, causing dissention and quarrels, or arguments over theology. The Lord warns us to stay away from people who cause division and exhibit toxic behaviors. Their toxic behavior creates unhealthy and harmful relationships that pull us away from the journey God wants us to be on.

**These are people the Lord warns us to stay away from:**

- **Those who do evil or have wicked friends:** *"Blessed is the man who <u>walks not</u> in the counsel of the wicked, nor stands in the way of sinners, nor sits in the seat of scoffers" (Psalm 1:1).*

- **Those lacking self-control:** *"<u>Make no friendship</u> with a man given to anger, nor go with a wrathful man, lest you learn his ways and entangle yourself in a snare" (Proverbs 22:24 – 25).*
  *Immoral people, especially those who claim to be Christians: "But now I am writing to you <u>not to associate with anyone who bears the name of brother</u> if he is guilty of sexual immorality or greed, or is an idolater, reviler, drunkard, or swindler—<u>not even to eat with such a one</u>" (1 Corinthians 5:11).*

  *"But understand this, that in the last days there will come times of difficulty. For people will be lovers of self, lovers of money, proud, arrogant, abusive, disobedient to their parents, ungrateful, unholy, heartless, unappeasable, slanderous, without self-control, brutal, not loving good, treacherous, reckless, swollen with conceit, lovers of pleasure rather than lovers of God, having the appearance of godliness, but denying its power. <u>Avoid such people</u>" (2 Timothy 3:1 – 5).*

- **People with perverted speech:** *"Discretion will watch over you, understanding will guard you, <u>delivering you from</u> the way of evil, <u>from men</u> of perverted speech, who forsake the paths of uprightness to walk in the ways of darkness" (Proverbs 2:11 – 13).*

- **People who gossip and slander:** *"Whoever goes about slandering reveals secrets; therefore, <u>do not associate</u> with a simple babbler" (Proverbs 20:19).*

- **People prone to jealousy and selfish ambition**: *"For where jealousy and selfish ambition exist, there will be disorder and every vile practice" (James 3:16).*

- **Those who claim to be Christians but do not display the character of a Christian, or who have wrong teaching**:  *"<u>Do not be unequally yoked with unbelievers</u>. For what partnership has righteousness with lawlessness? Or what fellowship has light with darkness?" (2 Corinthians 6:14).*
  *"Beware of false prophets, who come to you in sheep's clothing but inwardly are ravenous wolves. <u>You will recognize them by their fruits</u>" (Matthew 7:15 – 16)*

## Questions to Ponder

44.1) Are there people in your life who exhibit the previously mentioned traits? If yes, list them.

44.2) Based on your list, and the scriptures above, should you reevaluate your Q chart? Are there changes that you are <u>unwilling</u> to make in your relationships?

## Associating with People to Witness

Jesus commands you to share the Gospel with all nations, not to make the world your friend. It can be tempting to bring someone into your circle of friends, thinking your positive influence will lead them to Christ. Unfortunately, Scripture warns us that this is not the case:

*Do not be deceived: "Bad company ruins good morals." (1 Corinthians 15:33)*

*You therefore, beloved, knowing this beforehand, take care that you are not carried away with the error of lawless people and lose your own stability. (2 Peter 3:17)*

Imagine, you are out for a walk and see a filthy dog. It is caked in mud, mangy, half its hair missing, and covered in flees. The dog is dying. With compassion, you bring the dog into your home and try to clean it up. You drench it in water, removing enough of the dirt that it encourages you to keep trying. You grab a clean white rag to remove the mud, and you attempt to remove the clumps of earth matted into the dog's fur and skin. The rag picks up dirt and moves it around but never truly gets the dog clean, and the rag becomes soiled. You wash the rag, but it is no longer white; now it is stained a grey-brown color. You apply a heavy-duty shampoo to the dog's fur, but it seeps into his sores, and he yelps and runs off. He loved the attention and tolerated the water, but he never desired to be clean. When the process hit a sore spot, anger and fear made the life-saving bath seem threatening.

In the above illustration the **dog is like a sinner** who needs Christ, filthy from sin, and in pain from deep wounds in his heart. The **water is like the Word of God** that you witness to the sinner. As it flows over the sinner, it gives hope and opens a door to God's healing. **The white rag represents your heart.** You let the sinner into your heart and life, hoping your godliness will be the influence that makes the difference. The sinner loves the attention, taking full advantage of it. You realize the filth embedded deep in him and tell the sinner he needs a relationship with the Lord—the shampoo. His flesh burns with fear and anger, and he leaves. You can only clean up the surface appearance. **Only the Lord can destroy the flesh and change a heart.** Meanwhile, the sinner's influence, words, and manipulation leave your heart stained.

## The Takeaway

- We are supposed to share the Word, our testimony, and God's love with those in the world.

- Because of our sin nature, we must be diligent to protect what and who we allow to influence us.

- **We cannot make another righteous**, but they can influence us with evil.

- We represent God, but it is His job to draw people, save their soul, and change their heart.

- The Lord gives us discernment about who we should witness to and how.

## Purity in Relationship

*Who shall ascend the hill of the Lord? And who shall stand in his holy place? <u>He who has clean hands and a pure heart</u>, who does not lift up his soul to what is false and does not swear deceitfully. (Psalm 24:3 – 4)*

One of the greatest temptations facing us is sexual temptation. It manifests in a variety of ways: lusting over another, watching sexual content in entertainment, sex outside of marriage, multiple or same-sex partners, or adultery. Because every sexual sin begins in our mind, this is our focus.

*But I say to you that everyone who looks at a woman with lustful intent has already committed adultery with her in his heart. (Matthew 5:28)*

Your sin begins the moment you look at salacious material or let your mind wander into titillating fantasies. It is the same as if you commit the acts you are fantasizing about. To protect your relationships, you must first guard your mind's purity.

*To the pure, all things are pure, but to the defiled and unbelieving, nothing is pure; but both their minds and their consciences are defiled. (Titus 1:15)*

*For this is the will of God, your sanctification: that you abstain from sexual immorality; that each one of you know how to control his own body in holiness and honor, not in the passion of lust like the Gentiles who do not know God; that no one transgress and wrong his brother in this matter, because the Lord is an avenger in all these things, as we told you beforehand and solemnly warned you. <u>For God has not called us for impurity, but in holiness</u>. Therefore whoever disregards this, disregards not man but God, who gives his Holy Spirit to you. (1 Thessalonians 4:3 – 8)*

## Protecting Purity

It is easy to fall into the trap of sexual sin, especially in your mind. Therefore, it is important to protect purity of mind and body, and the integrity of your marriage or future marriage.

*How can a young man keep his way pure? By guarding it according to your word. (Psalm 119:9)*

The best guard against sexual sin is to **never give it room in your life**. Examine your motives and create reasonable boundaries. If you have a close friendship with someone of the opposite sex, consider how a new spouse may feel about that friendship. Protect your spouse; **do not tempt them to jealousy**.

Men and woman **do** need to interact in society, and this makes it important to create boundaries for your relationships. Examples of these boundaries may include not contacting anyone of the opposite gender privately or meeting with them alone behind closed doors. Create boundaries for your mind as well. Consider what people you meet with, where you go, and what you listen to or watch. Eliminate influences that cause your mind to wander where it should not.

## Questions to Ponder

44.3) Have you ever let someone into your inner circle because you wanted to "fix" them or be a positive influence in their lives? What was the result?

44.4) What temptations or influences cause your mind to wander to impure thoughts?

44.5) What can you do to keep your thoughts pure?

44.6) Are there any boundaries you should create? How will you enforce them?

# *Lesson 45 — Hidden Dangers*

> **IMPORTANT: Do not attempt to diagnose another person or yourself.**
>
> Often, people with destructive behavior experienced harm from their own trauma or dysfunctional relationships. However, do not attempt to diagnose another person or yourself. Instead, **use the terms in this lesson to identify the _toxic behaviors_ in yourself or others that harm your relationships.**

The following lessons deal with some of the **most** toxic relationship dynamics. **It can be difficult to identify these dynamics in a relationship when you're in the midst of it, and it can be hard to leave the toxic environment.** The information below can help you spot hidden manipulation, control, and enabling, as well as false thinking passed down from past generations. If you believe you are in a damaging relationship, please let your coach know. They have additional resources and can guide you to **professional help**.

## Codependency

Relationship is reciprocal by nature, meaning that both parties give to and receive from the relationship. Codependency distorts the reciprocal nature of a relationship. One person in the relationship meets his or her emotional needs (such as approval, worth, and value) by attempting to fix, enable, or mask another's unhealthy behavior. One is needy, the other needs to be needed. When Jesus fills all our needs, we are not dependent on another person to fill us. We become able to give to people out of an overflow of love. **Healthy relationships come from a desire to give oneself to another. Unhealthy relationships come from an attempt to fill a lack or a need.**

Codependent relationships prevent one or both parties from leading independent lives apart from the relationship. The relationship takes precedence over individual choices and pursuits. Codependency exists in most relationships where at least one of the people suffers from addiction, abuse, neglect, narcissism, or mental illness. The enabler sacrifices their individuality to care and cover for the dependent's physical or emotional issues.

Each person in a codependent relationship depends on the other's issues. Therefore, **healing one individual does not heal the relationship**. The strongholds no longer exist for the healed person, while the codependent continues to require that their needs to be met. **Both must heal or the relationship may not be sustainable.**

Codependency can exist between spouses, parents and children, friends, or coworkers. It is easy to live in denial about a codependent relationship, especially when you love the person or have made a significant investment in their life. Codependency may affect entire families, and toxic behaviors can be passed down to future generations. Codependent families often fear relying on outsiders, and they may hide or refuse to acknowledge problems in the family unit.

## Gaslighting and Manipulation

Manipulation in a relationship destroys the one being manipulated. **Gaslighting is a particularly detrimental form of manipulation used to control and twist the reality of the victim**. The manipulator will lie or skew the facts of a situation to their benefit or to defeat the other person's argument. A gaslighter may reject any answer you offer to defend the truth and argue with you to a point of exhaustion.

People who are gaslighted question their reality: *Did I remember that wrong?* The perpetrator gains control through a consistent misrepresenting of facts to confuse the victim, making them believe they are stupid or crazy.

A person who gaslights often displays passive-aggressive behaviors. They may put unrealistic expectations on the other person or engage in an ongoing conflict if the person disagrees. They might neglect a person's needs until they get their desired result. Ghosting, shunning, or ignoring are also forms of passive-aggression.

This kind of manipulation in a relationship keeps you spinning. Your accuser may act angry at himself for hurting you in one moment, and the next minute he is blaming you. The confusion this causes creates a belief that you are not good enough. You may even begin to question, "What is wrong with me?" Not able to find the answers, you reject yourself and begin to lean on other people, including your abuser, to know how to be.

**Healthy people communicate to be understood and to understand others.** A gaslighter only seeks to prove that he is right and refuses to acknowledge a different perspective. Gaslighting feeds on a person's fear of the manipulator's rejection and desire for their approval.

The following lists do not diagnose any mental illness or disorder.

## Signs of Codependency

*In the following lists*, **note all frequent or recurring signs** *in your relationships. If you feel unsafe, seek immediate help. Your coach has resources to help you.*

**Do you, or does someone in your life:**

- Spend all your energy meeting a person's needs and/or take responsibility for their happiness
- "Love" people that you can pity and rescue
- Feel trapped in a relationship
- Make most or all decisions
- Often rely on someone to decide for you
- Do most of the work to keep peace in a relationship
- Struggle to identify your feelings, or minimize, deny, or lie about how you feel
- Fear rejection or abandonment, or feel rejected if someone refuses your offer to help
- Engage in passive-aggressive behavior and/or consistent negativity
- Seek a sense of security and safety in someone else
- Hesitate to trust people
- Suffer low self-esteem or feelings of guilt or shame, or compare yourself with others

- Have difficulty saying "No"
- Struggle to sacrifice your own needs to please another
- Take responsibility for another person's wrong actions (i.e., apologizing for them, hiding their mistakes, or letting them off the hook)
- Defend and depend on the relationship, even at personal cost, believing it to be a selfless act
- Act over-sensitive or defensive in response to another's thoughts or feelings
- Violate boundaries, dictating the choices another person makes
- Have difficulty adjusting to change

## Signs of Being Gaslighted

**Do you:**

- Have difficulty deciding because you do not trust yourself to make right choices
- Feel you lost yourself, or you remember yourself as a different person from who you are now
- Feel as if you cause another's misery
- Second-guess yourself, feel confused, or question your sanity
- Doubt things occurred the way you remember them or question your reality
- Often get accused of being too sensitive, wrong, insane, emotional, or overreacting
- Lie or make excuses because of fear of being criticized, attacked, or ridiculed
- Feel wrong and inadequate ("I should be a better spouse/friend/etc.")
- Apologize even when you feel you were wronged
- Fear something is wrong or threatening but cannot identify it
- Make excuses for another person's behavior

### Questions to Ponder

45.1) Thinking about past relationships and your childhood family, do you recognize any of the signs of codependency? State which relationship and give examples.

45.2) Thinking about current relationships, do you recognize any of the signs of codependency? State which relationship and give examples.

45.3) Do you recognize any sign that someone may be gaslighting you? Explain.

45.4) Give past and current examples of when you have been gaslighted.

45.5) Do you see yourself gaslighting others? Who do you gaslight and how? Give examples.

*If you are in a manipulative or toxic relationship, **speak to your coach. He or she has additional resources available** for you and may direct you to professional help if needed.*

# *Lesson 46 — Dysfunction in the Family*

## The Dysfunctional Family Dynamic

When a family member has a mental illness, struggles with addiction, or is a narcissist, psychopath, or sociopath, it leads to a dysfunctional home environment. While these disorders may be different, the resulting dysfunction is similar. **Leave it to a professional to diagnose a mental disorder.** However, if you recognize the dynamics mentioned in this lesson in your current or childhood family, **seek the counsel of a mental health professional trained to deal with these disorders and the resulting trauma.**

Children growing up in a home with dysfunction may become adults who struggle with relationship issues. They often cannot figure out why they suffer from anxiety, depression, or other emotional symptoms. The following are lists of traits and roles commonly found in this dysfunctional family dynamic. **The level of dysfunction in the family depends on the degree of mental illness or abuse.** No family or relationship is the same as any other.

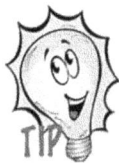

> Many people who were in abusive relationships , especially in their childhood families end up in similar abusive relationships in adulthood. It is an environment they understand how to live in. They develop a subconscious belief that they deserve the abuse.
>
> Often their **abuser defines love in a way that benefits the abuser and neglects the needs of the abused**. If this is you, it is vital to look at God's perspective of your value and love. It is difficult to break free from lies that you have spent your entire life believing. Submit these things to the Lord and have patience as He changes your heart to accept the truth.

## Healthy vs. Unhealthy Family Roles

**Members of a healthy family are interdependent.** They assume roles within the **family community**, but these roles change as a child develops and different circumstances arise. This is a normal part of development, giving the child needed skills to live as an independent adult. There is no threat to the family dynamic when roles change, a family member dies, or a child leaves to start their own family.

**In the dysfunctional family, roles are co-dependent and more rigid.** Children bury part of their personality to stay in their role. This stifles emotional development and prevents learning healthy adult skills, such as coping with emotions and resolving conflicts. The dysfunctional family functions as **one entity, the family itself, not as individuals in a family community**. A person's role may change only if it meets the needs of the family. Someone leaving their role leaves a gap, which threatens the family's stability. Think of this family as one body, one individual. A person leaving or changing roles is like cutting out a major organ. It cripples the functioning ability of the family unit.

## The Narcissistic Family

**Narcissism is a rare diagnosis, but the impact of narcissistic abuse is not rare.** Narcissism is a condition defined by a lack of empathy, an exaggerated belief in one's own self-importance, and the inability to admit wrongdoing. The narcissist proudly displays these beliefs in arrogant, patronizing, and demanding thoughts and actions. Narcissists manipulate others, thirst for approval and control, and are remarkably selfish. They **may play the victim** or seem untouchable.

Sometimes narcissistic behavior falls short of NPD (Narcissistic Personality Disorder). Any form or degree of narcissism or antisocial personality disorder creates an abusive environment that negatively impacts families. Bree Bonchay, LCSW, wrote a medically reviewed article in which he estimates narcissistic abuse affects half of the U.S. population in some way.[1]

Narcissistic abuse in the home creates a devastating family dynamic. Many adults suffer mental and emotional disorders resulting from the severe emotional abuse they endured as children, and **many find themselves in recovery programs**. The behaviors developed in a narcissistic family may transfer generationally, even if the children do not become narcissists. If you live in or come from a dysfunctional home, it is important to identify these toxic behaviors.

In this environment, children **must comply with the family narrative and value system or face rejection** from the family. The narcissist treats others as abnormal, like there is something wrong with them. This is manipulation. He creates insecurities and exploits people's strongholds to enforce control. The narcissist expects others to submit to his authority, even if it is wrong or abusive. He can read people's emotions and anticipate their responses, and he uses this information to guilt, shame, or coerce compliance. **Gaslighting is a favorite tool of the narcissist.**

Feelings of safety and security are absent in the home when a family member has narcissistic tendencies. Mistakes and accidents bring condemnation, whether or not a family member deserves guilt or admits his wrong. The family must hide abuse, often believing they are at fault for the abuse. Neglect and mistreatment create an atmosphere of continual fear in the home, but in public, the family puts on a good show, denying the truth of the life they are living, fearing the narcissist's ridicule, shame, and rage.

People living in a home with a true narcissist have difficulty escaping the environment without intervention. They usually do not have strong personalities, as the narcissist will work to prevent anyone close to them from having more power and influence than they do. When someone does stand up to a narcissist by establishing boundaries, the narcissist pushes or manipulates the boundaries, exhausting anyone trying to live free from their control.

**Narcissistic families often exhibit pseudomutuality**, which means that although the family is broken, they **appear** unified and tight-knit to the outside world. Disagreements become divisive and force family members to choose sides. Shame and ridicule are the cost of choosing the wrong side. Children may feel forced to choose between parents, siblings, or other family members who do not side with the narcissist. Only the narcissist may express their feelings, especially rage, discounting dissenting opinions and feelings and training others to suppress their emotional responses. In this kind of family, respecting one person requires that you disrespect another to keep up appearances. Love and respect are not available to everyone at once; some earn praise while others are shamed. The family roles in a narcissistic family change with the situation to maintain the family dynamic but not to benefit the individual.

---

[1] "Narcissistic Abuse Affects Over 158 Million People in the U.S.," *PsychCentral*, https://psychcentral.com/lib/narcissistic-abuse-affects-over-158-million-people-in-the-u-s/.

## Traits of the Dysfunctional Family

- Children lack emotional access to parents. They do not feel heard, seen, or nurtured. Parents are judgmental and critical of their children.

- A narcissist may pit children against each other and compare them to one another. The parent may favor one child while another takes the brunt of his anger and frustration until the roles change. Siblings may grow up protecting one another, but more often they feel an emotional disconnect from one another.

- Children lack boundaries, or the boundaries change as the whim of the parent changes.

- Children learn negative messages about themselves through their parents' words and actions. They believe they are not good enough or are somehow defective. They believe they must earn their value by what they do instead of being valued for who they are.

- Children lack guidance, love, and direction from their parents. Instead, they serve the parents' emotional or physical needs, creating a distorted view of what love is.

- The family lacks respect for physical and emotional boundaries. No one has a right to privacy. Children learn unclear personal boundaries and never understand, even into adulthood, that family does not have the right to violate their privacy.

- Family members who cannot discuss their feelings experience multiple emotional issues. They believe the others consider their feelings unimportant, and they are too sensitive. The narcissist projects their own feelings onto others, and everyone else must repress their emotions, processing them in damaging ways.

- Family members experience emotional, psychological, and often physical abuse.

- The family keeps secrets. They must hide profound pain from the outside world and pretend nothing is wrong. The secrets become their reality.

- The family must maintain an image of perfection. Everything must seem better than it is. They worry about what friends, family, and neighbors will think of them.

- Effective communication skills are nonexistent in any sort of conflict. Unless presented as rage, there is no direct communication of an issue. It is easier to talk about another than to confront them, so the family often communicates through triangulation. This is when one person tells information about another to a third person, knowing, eventually, the person being talked about will hear it.

- Passive-aggressive behaviors create tension and an inability to trust other family members with your heart.

## Roles in the Dysfunctional Family

Families suffering from addiction, mental illness, narcissism, and other forms of dysfunction have distinct family roles. Note that **seeing yourself in one of these roles does not necessarily indicate the type of dysfunction in your family**. Not all roles are present in all families.

A narcissistic parent's expectations may **force a child into a specific role**, or a child may **take on a specific role as a coping skill** or may **assume multiple roles**. Children suffering emotional abuse, like all children, need the attention and validation that are lacking in a dysfunctional environment. The family role that a child plays may continue into adulthood if he does not learn and apply healthy coping skills.

### Key roles in the dysfunctional family

Read the two lists that follow, describing toxic behaviors and family roles. Note each role or sign that you recognize in your current or past relationships. Then answer the questions at the end.

- **The Focal Point** – The person, often a parent, to whom the family devotes their attention and energy. This role usually exists in a family where one or both parents have addiction, narcissism, psychopathy, or another personality disorder.

- **Orbiting Parent** – In a home where the focal point is one parent, the orbiting parent is the spouse. The children may be sympathetic as they see her as being treated unfairly by the other parent. Even so, the orbiting parent is too busy "orbiting" or appeasing the focal point to fully meet the children's needs.

- **The Golden Child** – The golden child can do no wrong. The focal point displays this child as a reflection of himself. He sees something about this child which gives him "bragging rights." The golden child believes that his value comes from what he does, and he perceives people less accomplished as having little value.

- **The Scapegoat Child** – The scapegoat is the child who does nothing right. He is the "bad seed" or "black sheep" of the family. He receives the brunt of a parent's anger, unrelenting blame, and **suffers humiliation in front of other family members**. The scapegoat is authentic and truthful about the family's issues and unjust behaviors. They may mean well but often act out in anger or rebellion in response to the injustice. The other family members expect the scapegoat to care about the family's needs, while treating them as if they have no needs of their own. Scapegoats do not receive the credit they deserve for their achievements, and they can never live up to their parents' expectations. They often have a deep-seated belief that they are incapable, worthless, and unloved.

- **Invisible/Lost Child** – This child is ignored because the parents are focused on their own issues and other children. The lost child **does not receive praise or blame** but is forgotten or treated as if they are invisible. Parents may care for the child's basic needs, but there is no investment in their life. These children learn basic life skills by watching siblings, and they become very independent. Believing they have no voice, they withdraw into their own little world. Lost children often struggle to feel like they fit in. They feel lonely, invisible, unloved, and unvalued.

**Secondary Roles in dysfunctional families** (Secondary roles may pair with key roles.)

- **The Dependent** – Dependents fall into a deep pit of substance abuse or dysfunction and face the most obvious challenges to recovery. The problem child, acting out in rebellion, is often a dependent. Everyone, including the dependent, realizes his behaviors must change. The family alters their behaviors to accommodate the dependent's lifestyle by enabling them and lying for them, willingly or unwillingly. Some may react by cutting off all contact with the dependent, which can change the entire family dynamic. The dependent must identify their unhealthy behavior and thought patterns to recover.

- **The Mastermind** – The mastermind is a manipulator and opportunist, often using coercion to get what he wants. This may is often a narcissist or he may be a dependent, using manipulation to continue or hide his substance use. Masterminds are self-absorbed, abusive, and driven by entitlement. A mastermind will intentionally confuse the family members to hide the truth about himself and his abuse. He will use and manipulate the rest of the family's dysfunction to his own benefit. He observes each person's behaviors and engages their dysfunctional role at will to achieve his intended purpose. He may create intentional conflict among family members to serve his interests. He knows how to use his charm to manipulate both the children and adults in the family. Masterminds may rebel or act like the scapegoat, engaging in their own form of misbehavior. They may take advantage of the caretaker's nature or use another enabler to get what they want. A mastermind is difficult to understand. His actions are despicable, but he creates chaos and takes advantage of people and opportunities, often to meet his own neglected needs.

- **Flying Monkey** – Like the flying monkeys in The Wizard of Oz, this enabler reports on and torments non-compliant family members—anyone who contradicts the "focal point," or anyone considered a threat to the family. Their unwavering loyalty to the family makes them easy to manipulate. The focal point uses the flying monkey's own issues to manipulate her to perpetrate abuse on his targeted victims through gaslighting, threats, guilt, shame, rejection, or violence. This clears the focal point of all wrongdoing. While the focal point is manipulating the flying monkey to do his dirty work, he may also be manipulating the target by acting selfless or as a temporary martyr to gain deeper trust and commitment from them.

- **The Mascot** – The mascot is the family joker, using humor and antics to relieve the stress in the home. Their jokes are often insensitive or immature. They tend to be the center of attention and popular because of their "class clown" antics. Mascots cannot deal with the feelings of powerlessness that arise from conflict, violence, anger, or other negative family situations. They use humor to communicate repressed emotions; to hide deep insecurity; to avoid conflict rather than address issues; and to escape difficult emotions like pain, grief, anger, or fear. Humor becomes the mascot's identity. She has many superficial friends but is unable to sustain a deep relationship. She cannot let anyone see the person behind her jester mask. The mascot stays too busy to stop and think, attempting to avoid the depression and anxiety that come in the quiet. She may have difficulty concentrating, leading to problems in school or at a job. The mascot is a people-pleaser, so her adult relationships are often codependent.

- **Caretaker** – This family member is an enabler who covers up or makes excuses for the issues of the addict/narcissist. She becomes the family martyr, taking care of the addict/narcissist's responsibilities, and protecting him from the consequences of his actions or taking them upon herself. The caretaker seeks to be the emotional rescuer for the rest of the family but neglects her own emotional support. She expresses sensitivity to emotion and often seems calm and caring. A caretaker bases her self-worth and identity on her ability to help the family. She shows her concern with nurturing support, listening, consoling, protecting, and advising family members, yet her efforts to save the family enforce each person's codependent roles. Caretakers are people-pleasers and problem-fixers—that is, they solve everyone's problems but their own. They have everyone's answers, but do not know how to care for themselves. They give love, but do not know how to receive it, and they may push genuine love away. Caretakers often experience trauma bonding with the narcissist. In adulthood, they often have **highly toxic codependent relationships, which become one-sided and abusive**. They tend to become everyone's doormat.

- **Hero** – The hero wants to present a "normal" family appearance. This is the perfectionist who, like the caretaker, covers up family secrets. The hero takes responsibility for the family image and becomes the true mask of a dysfunctional family. Heroes suppress their own emotions so much that they are unable to experience most emotions at all. Their insecurity drives them to be accomplished and successful, seeking achievement in any form possible. The hero is often the older sibling, but not always. The hero is stuck in his ways, the self-appointed responsible one, who expects perfection—from himself and others—to maintain the family image. He appears to be the most successful, "together" person in the family, but accomplishments do not satisfy his needs. Heroes suffer from their high expectations and stress levels and develop major control issues to avoid feeling guilt and shame from failure. They place blame on other family members for their family's issues creating volatile relationships in the home, but sometimes people outside of the home bear the brunt of the blame. Their family's problems become the fault of whoever benefits the hero's narrative.

## Questions to Ponder

46.1) Do the people in your family (whether now or in the past) have roles that are interdependent or codependent? Do the roles respect individuality? Explain your answers.

46.2) Do you recognize any of the traits of a dysfunctional family from your childhood family or other past relationships? Explain and give examples.

46.3) Do you recognize any of the traits of a dysfunctional family in your current relationships? Explain and give examples.

46.4) Thinking about your childhood family and past relationships, can you see yourself or other family members in dysfunctional family "roles"? Explain and give examples.

46.5) Thinking about your current family dynamic, do you see yourself or other family members that fit in a specific role? Explain and give examples.

*If you are stuck in a manipulative or toxic relationship, <u>speak to your coach for more help.</u>*

# Lesson 47 — Insist on Healthy Relationships

Movies and television shows often depict people with personality disorders as mass murderers capable of an insane amount of harm. This makes entertaining fiction, but actual people rarely act this way. In real life, people suffering from personality disorders may not show the outward signs you might expect. For example, a covert narcissist may act passive, give fake apologies, be quiet, or seem like the victim. A psychopath **may** be violent but **will** cause emotional and psychological harm. Having multiple disorders may compound a person's dysfunction.

It is important to recognize damaging behaviors, but do not make your own diagnoses. Someone who exhibits any of these behaviors needs professional, godly help from a therapist **trained to deal with these disorders**. A person without training **cannot diagnose them or fix them**. Remember, most people's dysfunctional behaviors arise from significant pain and insecurity. Please do not try to change them. Instead, examine their behavior and **change your own** to protect yourself from harmful situations.

## Protecting Yourself from Dangerous Relationships

**Instead of focusing on the poor behavior of another, focus on yourself.** You cannot control what people do, but you can control how you respond to their words and actions. **Confidence in your own identity, loving yourself, and knowing healthy relationship dynamics** can prevent a negative or dysfunctional person from abusing you.

### Shame

A person riddled with shame is a prime target for manipulation and abuse. This is why it is vital to know your value and identity as a child of God. You cannot have confidence to step out of dysfunction if a little voice inside you whispers that you deserve the abuse. You cannot fight the lies of dysfunction without a healthy love for yourself. Remind yourself of the truth found in God's Word: The guilts and shame of the past no longer belong to you. Love the person you are in Christ, love the new creation you are becoming, and have confidence that God will finish the work He started in you. Know without doubt that you are worth treating well because your creator says you are. **Love yourself enough to stand up for yourself. The way people treat you matters as much as how you treat them.** Their words do not define you. Stand firm in the truth.

> *Fear not, for you will not be ashamed; be not confounded, for you will not be disgraced;*
> *for you will forget the shame of your youth, and the reproach of your widowhood*
> *you will remember no more. (Isaiah 54:4)*

> *Bless the Lord, O my soul, and forget not all his benefits, who forgives all your iniquity,*
> *who heals all your diseases, who redeems your life from the pit, who crowns you with*
> *steadfast love and mercy. (Psalm 103:2 – 4)*

Shame, especially when it has been embedded in your heart since childhood, is difficult to overcome. Like everything else in recovery, it is a process. Speak with your coach about areas of shame you still hold on to. Look for any problematic thinking patterns that remain and remind yourself daily of who you are and who you are becoming. The more you bring lies into the light, the less power they have.

# Understand Healthy Relationships

Understanding healthy relationships helps you identify how people should fit into your life. Regardless of the relationship, every person should treat you with respect.

| Healthy Relationship | Unhealthy Relationship |
|---|---|
| ➤ Each person values the relationship equally. | ➤ The relationship feels one-sided. |
| ➤ Each person respects the other as an individual outside the relationship. | ➤ At least one person feels they may not have a life outside the relationship. |
| ➤ Neither person feels other friendships threaten the relationship. | ➤ Jealousy causes control or manipulation of the other person's friendships. |
| ➤ Each person supports the other's hobbies, interests, and other pursuits. | ➤ One tries to control the decisions of the other or makes all the decisions for them. |
| ➤ Each person shares their lives, interests, and pain. If you know another fully, you know and care about what hurts them. | ➤ They share common interests and activities but have no desire or ability to share the deep matters of their heart or their pain. |
| ➤ Both people are honest and truthful. | ➤ Lies and manipulation are common. |
| ➤ Each person is free to express an opposing viewpoint. | ➤ One or both people ridicule and dismiss opposing viewpoints. |
| ➤ Both people trust one another with their flaws and innermost secrets. | ➤ Both people put up walls to guard their hearts. |
| ➤ Each person bears the other's burdens and considers the best interests of the other. | ➤ One person dismisses the other's needs, expecting his own needs to take precedence. |
| ➤ Each person has access to material and financial assets. | ➤ Money is a means to control and manipulate. |
| ➤ Each person overflows love into the other. | ➤ The relationship is built on need, not love. |
| ➤ Both people treat each other with kindness and understanding. | ➤ One or both people treat the other with contempt and ridicule. |
| ➤ Each person is gracious, overlooking the other's faults and mistakes and helping them overcome. | ➤ One or both people believe that a person can never be better than their mistakes and faults. |
| ➤ Communication is open and honest and allows a healthy expression of feelings. | ➤ Those in the relationship cannot communicate their feelings without worrying about insults and ridicule. |
| ➤ Both people feel heard when sharing their thoughts and feelings. | ➤ At least one person feels like the other never hears them, or like their words do not matter. |
| ➤ Both people can offer and receive correction in a disagreement, stick to the subject, have self-control, admit wrongdoing, and problem-solve to find resolution. | ➤ In a disagreement, one person faces ridicule and condemnation as the other attempts to cover up wrongdoing and shut down the conversation. The goal is not resolution. |
| ➤ Both are walking together with the Lord. | ➤ The people in the relationship are on different spiritual paths. |
| ➤ In a marital relationship, each person feels safe and comfortable with the sexual activity. | ➤ One person in the marriage pressures or forces the other to engage in sexual activity they are not comfortable with. |

If your relationship(s) has a few unhealthy characteristics, you can work to correct damaging behaviors. However, when a person is **unwilling to communicate, recognize, or change their behavior**, it may be time to end the relationship. When you cannot distance yourself from a relationship, you must set boundaries.

## Boundaries

Boundaries are not a means of control or manipulation. Boundary-setting is not a passive-aggressive behavior that withholds communication, finances, or love until the other person complies with your will. You are not forcing someone to agree with you or do things your way. Boundaries protect you from abuse. Creating distance or boundaries gives you the space you need to heal.

Creating healthy boundaries in a relationship involves **defining clear rules** about what you will not allow in your life and **consistent enforcement** of those rules. You should implement some boundaries with everyone you interact with. Make the rules fit your circumstances. Bear in mind that it is in our flesh to push boundaries and bend rules. **Bendable rules mean breached boundaries.**

Manipulators attempt to find ways around boundaries. They might try to convince you that you are wrong for creating boundaries in the first place, or trick you into dropping boundaries altogether. You may need separation to establish healthy boundaries. If you cannot cut off contact, create distance and limit interaction. Prepare to walk out of the room or stop communication the moment a person violates one of your rules.

## Essential Rules for Every Relationship

**"You will respect me."** Tolerate no ridicule, name-calling, insults, gaslighting, manipulation, guilt trips, or false accusations. End the conversation immediately.

**"You will respect my time. I am not obligated to your time frame."** Do not feel guilty about making someone wait for your schedule to be free. You can respect their desires so long as you realize that your life does not revolve around their schedule.

**"You will respect my words. When I say no, the answer is no."** Do not allow others to pressure you to do something that violates your boundaries or morals, or that makes you uncomfortable. It is okay to refuse to help someone. You know the amount of responsibility you can handle. It is your right to consider your own needs.

**"You will respect my privacy."** Do not allow another to violate your online or offline privacy. Your home, belongings, conversations, body, and life are your business. Spying on you, following you, asking others about you, going through your phone or journals, or talking/gossiping about you are never acceptable behavior.

**"You will respect my choices."** It is not your responsibility to meet another's expectations, (except perhaps when performing your job, or when you choose to commit to a responsibility). Set reasonable expectations for yourself and live by those standards. You are free to make your own choices in life.

**"If you have a problem with me, come to me directly."** Triangulation is not acceptable. If someone takes issue with you, they should address it with you and not gossip to another about the issue.

<u>Questions to Ponder</u>

47.1) Do you feel shame from any of the relationships in your life? Which words or actions make you feel shameful, and who causes those feelings?

47.2) Looking at the traits of healthy and unhealthy relationships, how do you feel about the quality of your close relationships?

47.3) Examine the relationships with the greatest impact on your life. Are there unhealthy behaviors in these relationships? List them.

47.4) You should have healthy boundaries in every relationship. Which relationships consistently violate healthy boundaries?

47.5) Do you feel trapped in a relationship with mental or physical abuse? Do you feel unheard, ridiculed, or gaslighted? Describe these relationships.

47.6) Abusive relationships require stronger boundaries. Review the information _on the next pages_ about establishing and enforcing healthy boundaries. Then make a plan.

*If you believe you are in a toxic mentally or physically abusive relationship,*
*ask your coach to direct you to professional help.*

Obviously, **it is easier to avoid a toxic or abusive relationship** than to deal with one you are already in. How you handle this depends on your situation. If a person's abuse is a stumbling block to you following the Lord or His will for your life, choose the Lord first. **The next few pages give guidelines to establish healthy boundaries in relationships.**
*Do not think that I have come to bring peace to the earth. I have not come to bring peace, but a sword. For I have come to set a man against his father, and a daughter against her mother, and a daughter-in-law against her mother-in-law. And a person's enemies will be those of his own household. Whoever loves father or mother more than me is <u>not worthy of me</u>, and whoever loves son or daughter more than me is <u>not worthy of me</u>. And whoever does not take his cross and follow me is <u>not worthy of me</u>. Whoever finds his life will lose it, and <u>whoever loses his life for my sake will find it</u>. (Matthew 10:34 – 39)*

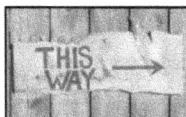

| THIS WAY → | Your coach has additional resources to help you learn, establish, and enforce healthy boundaries. |
|---|---|

## Enforcing Boundaries

In a dysfunctional or narcissistic family dynamic, **your boundaries are seen as a threat and will be met with resistance.** Those threatened by your boundaries may attempt to manipulate you, **dictate your choices**, or **isolate** you from people who speak a narrative different from theirs. **They may ridicule you, lay guilt on you, say they cannot live without you, or warn that they will do something drastic if you leave.** They may **intimidate**, **threaten**, or make it seem like **you are in the wrong.** If an abuser ignores or encroaches upon your boundaries, you must enforce your boundary with consequences. However, sometimes a broken person with a repentant heart is working with God to change toxic behaviors. As their behavior changes, you may modify the original boundaries.

**Here are the key things to remember when setting boundaries:**

❖ **God defines you; the abuser does not.** Do not allow anyone to tell you who you are or define your character or your intelligence. An abuser may accuse you of something they are doing. For example, if they are gossiping, they may accuse you of spreading gossip. Do not allow anyone to define your actions or motives.

❖ **You are not on trial. Do not give a defense.** An abuser may scrutinize your actions and lob false accusations at you. Do not allow intimidation to cause you to second guess what you know is true or right. **In a relationship in which you do not trust your heart to an abuser, you do not owe him an explanation or need to justify your thoughts, feelings, or actions.** The abuser gains a sense of power and control when he pushes your buttons. He feels superior when dissecting your perceived poor qualities. He may judge every word you say while accusing you of being judgmental. **You cannot win in this scenario.** Refuse to take part. Keep your mind focused on truth and stop accusations and insults immediately by walking away.

❖ **You have the power!** You have control and power over your choices, your feelings, and your thoughts. You are allowed to feel your feelings, think your own thoughts, and make your own choices. Even if your choices are bad, they are your mistakes to make. A controlling person tries to disempower you by making you feel bad for your choices or insisting you do things their way. Remember, you are an individual with your own mind. Other people will not experience the consequences of your actions; **you will**. Make your choices based on what you believe is best for your own life with the Lord's leading.

❖ **Avoid sharing personal information.** An abuser loses any right to details about your life or feelings. **They will use this information against you.** Keep conversations to mundane topics like the weather or news. If you must share a decision, avoid discussing the reason behind your choice. An abuser may draw you in with a need. Be unavailable. You do not need to explain yourself. Stay uninvolved. When drama or gossip is the topic being discussed, do not share your advice, opinions, or problem-solve. An abusive person may use your goodwill to violate your boundaries or to drag you into another's personal drama.

❖ **Plan to avoid manipulation.** Keep separate finances. Stop gaslighting and turn it back on them with the truth. Do not allow them to drive you to anger. Walk away from the "silent treatment." Plan a response to a manipulator's **FOG tactic** (fear, obligation, and guilt), which he may use against you. **Plan and practice** ways to enforce your boundaries and responses to the person's manipulation tactics.

**Use the following suggestions to prepare yourself to enforce boundaries:**

❖ **Prevent manipulation.** When you set boundaries, your abuser will pull out all the stops. Manipulation can seem like your own thoughts, making it exceedingly difficult to identify. The abuser may minimize your feelings while blaming you for how much you have hurt them. They act innocent, as if **they are the victim** of your anger, or accuse you of being sensitive or emotional.

To help identify manipulation, use the acrostic **FOG: Fear, Obligation, and Guilt**. This is a tactic an abuser uses **to fog your mind and make it difficult for you to see the truth**. For example, an abuser may cause you to worry about him or the future (fear). He may make you feel obligated to speak to him or treat him differently (obligation). He may try to make you feel wrong for standing up for yourself or attack your perceived character flaws (guilt). This tactic is effective against people struggling with insecurity and shame. **Have confidence** in the Lord as a just protector, **believe in your identity in Christ**, and **stick with your plan** to escape the harm your abuser causes.

**These are the key points to remember to prevent manipulation:**

- Identify the manipulation the abuser uses.

- Remind yourself that your boundaries are not up for discussion.

- Remember to keep your emotions out of any conversation. Be diligent to observe your abuser's behavior and do not take it on yourself.

- Do not engage a question designed to lure you into a trap. Keep conversations brief.

- Do not talk about your personal choices or engage in conversations about their choices.

- If the abuser gives you the silent treatment, stop trying to communicate with them.

- Journal everything. Know what they said and how it made you feel. Keep records so you know the truth and are not manipulated by gaslighting attempts.

❖ **Remain steadfast.** An abuser attempts to test boundaries like a child seeing how far he can push a parent before getting a spanking. When you set boundaries, expect retaliation. You are in a battle for yourself. **If your borders are not solid, the abuser will breach them.** You are important, and you have a God-given purpose. Persevere. Do not give up on yourself or give in to the abuse.

❖ **Prepare your finances.** In a healthy marriage, you should take part in financial decisions and partake in the family income with your spouse. Separate your finances, however, if your spouse seeks to control your spending, spend all the money, or keep money from you. Let him have his own money and take responsibility for yours. Separating your finances prevents an abuser from manipulating you with money.

❖ **Keep focused on yourself, not your abuser.** Keep your thoughts focused on your God, your rules, and your power over yourself. Don't waste precious time trying to get your abuser to understand how he hurt you; your explanations will likely fall on deaf ears. You may want him to care about you, or maybe you seek validation, but only the Lord can show him the truth. If he twists everything you say or do to validate himself, he will never hear or see you correctly. Constant rejection can make anyone question their value. Stop allowing an abuser to rob you of your value with their indifference and waste your time with fruitless effort. **You cannot change them, but you can alter your response!**

❖ **Prepare your emotions.** Does your abuser bring out the worst in you? We often become like the people we are around, especially picking up their negative traits. Remember our story about the dog? **When you reflect the abuser's behaviors,** such as criticizing, angry outbursts, or contempt, **he will ridicule you for your behavior.** This removes attention from him and places it on your "bad character." Building an emotional resistance to his actions will stop this cycle. You must have confidence. God says who you are, not your abuser.

**Here are some key ways to master your emotions as you enforce your boundaries:**

- **Do not internalize negative traits an** abuser projects on you. Recognize them as lies. For example, you may display anger, but that does not mean you are an angry person.

- **Understand your abuser.** Learn why they are behaving this way. What is their behavior, or your response to it, providing them? Realize the problem is with them and not you.

- **Watch, listen, and do not react.** You must stay calm and keep your emotions detached from the situation. Make a conscious decision to view your abuser as if from a distance. Observe what he does, as well as your behavior and responses. What can you learn about yourself and your abuser? Can you see manipulation tactics? What does it tell you about his character or yours? (Ask your coach for additional resources).

- **Do not reciprocate.** If an abuser responds in anger, do not show anger. Remove yourself from the situation. If he insults you, do not absorb or return the insult. When he is nice, say thank you, but do not give more. **No reaction means he has nothing to manipulate.**

- **Direct the conversation** back to the truth.

- **Remember your gratitude** for the blessings the Lord has provided and the work he has done in your life and keep your joy.

- **Advocate for yourself** the way you would for any other abused person.

❖ **Boundaries need consequences.** If an abuser violates your boundaries, prepare a consequence. It is vital that you be consistent, or your boundaries are worthless. A consequence may be to end a phone conversation, discontinue communication, leave a situation, or call the police. It is **your right and obligation to yourself to exit a destructive interaction.** You do not need approval or permission to leave or end communication. Your wellbeing is at stake. If your actions to enforce your boundaries jeopardize your physical safety, you may need to find shelter or involve the authorities.

❖ **Use preplanned, practiced responses.** Note how your abuser gets to you, and plan how you will respond to the situation. If a pat answer does not end the manipulation, stop the conversation immediately. State simple responses in a matter-of-fact tone.

- "The Lord uses my failure for my good."

- "I am confident in my choice."

- "No, you are interrupting me."

- "No, you may not speak to me that way."

- "No, that is not true."

- "Stop, you are disrespecting me." (Or manipulating me, discounting my feelings, etc.)

- "This is not constructive; I am ending this conversation." (Give no further explanation.)

# Chapter Eighteen

## Conflict Resolution

# *Lesson 48 — Conflict*

The last chapter dealt with atypical situations found in serious dysfunction. **Conflict is not a dangerous concept in most situations.** In this chapter, we will learn about healthy conflict. First, let us review what we already learned.

- **Conflict** brings resolution and restoration. A **fight or quarrel** is a power struggle to prove your point, not a genuine attempt at reconciliation.

- **Search your heart** before engaging another in conflict. Is your anger justified? What is the other person's perspective? What could skew your perspective?

- **Go directly to the person** who sins against you and privately address the wrong. Do not seek validation of your emotions from a third party.

- **Be quick to address a matter** to give the devil no place to meddle in the situation. If someone has a problem with you, address the issue right away. As much as it depends on you, live at peace with everyone.

## Why Engage in Conflict?

The easiest way through any issue is straight ahead. Always address a problem right away. It may make you sick just thinking about conflict, but **buried problems fester; they do not go away**. They escalate in your mind, so any reminder of the transgression brings back every hurt feeling.

**Refusing to deal with an offense is unfair to you and to the one who offended you.** They may be unaware of their offense or be responding to a hurt you caused them. Regardless of how much you love the other person, running away or refusing to communicate leaves unresolved pain for everyone involved, causing bitterness.

## Agree to Disagree?

Have you ever heard someone say, "Let's just agree to disagree on this"? People think differently. Sometimes it is not worth breaking unity with another person to prove your point. This can be a good way to end frivolous arguments while respecting another's differences.

On the other hand, people often misuse "agreeing to disagree" to prevent someone with an opposing viewpoint from speaking their thoughts, to end uncomfortable conversations, to shift blame, or to avoid conflict altogether. This prevents ideas from being heard and **stops a conflict that may bring healing**. It is never okay to agree to disagree to avoid dealing with your wrongs or to allow another to avoid dealing with their wrongs toward you.

> ## Questions to Ponder
> **48.1) Do you notice a difference in the way you handle conflict now compared to the way you handled conflict before beginning your journey? Explain**

48.2) What problems do you still have with conflict?

48.3) How do you avoid conflict or agree to disagree to keep peace in a situation?

## To Judge or Not to Judge

When conflict arises, people may accuse you of judging them, or you may feel you are being judged. Perhaps the verse most taken out of context and misapplied is Matthew 7:1, "Judge not, that you be not judged." Sometimes we **must** judge another's actions. Misunderstandings clear up when you read further and in context with other passages of Scripture.

> *Judge not, that you be not judged. For with the judgment you pronounce you will be judged, and with the measure you use it will be measured to you. Why do you see the speck that is in your brother's eye, but do not notice the log that is in your own eye? Or how can you say to your brother, "Let me take the speck out of your eye," when there is the log in your own eye? You hypocrite, first take the log out of your own eye, and then you will see clearly to take the speck out of your brother's eye. Do not give dogs what is holy, and do not throw your pearls before pigs, lest they trample them underfoot and turn to attack you. ... Beware of false prophets, who come to you in sheep's clothing but inwardly are ravenous wolves. (Matthew 7:1 – 6, 15)*

How will you recognize the "wolves," "dogs," and "pigs" if you do not judge? When someone is in sin or harming you, **it is perfectly acceptable to judge their actions**. However, when you look at another through the lens of your strongholds, you cannot make a righteous judgment. **First, you must examine your own heart** to discover the truth.

- Did you "take the log out of your eye" by examining your own heart and motives?
- Take an honest look from the other person's perspective. Are they right?
- Is this a situation in which you should show understanding and grace?
- Does your perspective of the conflict seem out of character for the other person?
- Is this an ongoing issue or a simple mistake you can overlook? Not every situation requires confrontation.

## Right Judgment

Sometimes we **should** judge, and we **can** discern good and evil. However, right judgment of another's actions requires maturity in Christ.

- You must use discernment to judge righteously; do not base your judgement on appearances.
- You may judge a person's actions as right or wrong by God's standards.
- You are to judge those in the church and purge evil people from your inner circles.
- God judges those outside the church.

> *And his delight shall be in the fear of the Lord. He shall not judge by what his eyes see, or decide disputes by what his ears hear. (Isaiah 11:3)*

*I wrote to you in my letter not to associate with sexually immoral people—not at all meaning the sexually immoral of this world, or the greedy and swindlers, or idolaters, since then you would need to go out of the world. But now I am writing to you <u>not to associate</u> with anyone who bears <u>the name of brother</u> if he is guilty of sexual immorality or greed, or is an idolater, reviler, drunkard, or swindler—not even to eat with such a one. For what have I to do with judging outsiders? <u>Is it not those inside the church whom you are to judge?</u> God judges those outside. "<u>Purge the evil person from among you.</u>" (1 Corinthians 5:9 – 13)*

*For everyone who lives on milk is unskilled in the word of righteousness, since he is a child. But solid food <u>is for the mature</u>, for those who have <u>their powers of discernment trained by constant practice</u> to distinguish good from evil. (Hebrews 5:13 – 14)*

Do you ever wonder why in one verse are we told to judge some people, and in others we are told not to judge people? The difference is in **how** we judge them.

- We should not pass judgment on unbelievers.
- We must not judge people before checking our own heart (removing the log from our eye).
- Judging wrongly is when we speak evil against a brother (a fellow Christian).
- Right judgment is sincere, impartial, full of mercy, reasonable, gentle, and wise.
- You must not judge a weaker believer for **their lack of faith**.

*Therefore you have no excuse, O man, every one of you who judges. For in passing judgment on another you condemn yourself, <u>because you, the judge, practice the very same things</u>. (Romans 2:1)*

*Do not speak evil against one another, brothers. <u>The one who speaks against a brother or judges his brother, speaks evil</u> against the law and judges the law. But if you judge the law, you are not a doer of the law but a judge. There is only one lawgiver and judge, he who is able to save and to destroy. But who are you to judge your neighbor? (James 4:11 – 12)*

*But the wisdom from above is first pure, then peaceable, gentle, open to reason, full of mercy and good fruits, impartial and sincere. (James 3:17)*

*As <u>for the one who is weak in faith</u>, welcome him, but <u>not to quarrel over opinions</u>. (Romans 14:1)*

## Questions to Ponder

48.4) When have you judged another wrongly? Explain.

48.5) Do you tend to pass judgments on others based on what annoys you?

48.6) When have you judged someone for something that you yourself did/do?

48.7) What does it mean to not judge the world? ("For what have I to do with judging outsiders?")

48.8) Do you argue with or judge others if they hold a different opinion? If so, why?

## Engage in Conflict

Scripture tells us to reconcile **with the one who offended** us **and** with **those we have offended**. It is our responsibility to put forth genuine effort to resolve the issue, **regardless of who was at fault**. Our pride and anger often demand that a person come to us for resolution, but this is not God's way. We must take responsibility and resolve the issue in a timely manner. The longer a matter goes unresolved, the more difficult it is to resolve. The longer questions and misconceptions go unanswered, the more opportunity for vain imaginations to make an offense seem worse than it was.

*Bearing with one another and, if one has a complaint against another, forgiving each other; as the Lord has forgiven you, so you also must forgive.*
*(Colossians 3:13)*

*Be angry and do not sin; do not let the sun go down on your anger, and give no opportunity to the devil. (Ephesians 4:26 – 27)*

## When the Issue Is Against You

If you know someone holds an offense against you, examine your heart and see if you are in the wrong. Either way, go to the person and hear their heart on the matter. If you are in the wrong, apologize and repent. If you are confident your actions were right, do your best to help them understand the situation. Apologize for misunderstandings and your part in the offense. Do **not apologize or feel guilt** for a problem you did not create. People often project their guilt onto others when emotions are involved. Set feelings aside and focus on the truth of the situation. Put your best effort into resolution; it is the other person's choice to receive or reject what you say.

*If possible, so far as it depends on you, live peaceably with all. (Romans 12:18)*

**Some things to remember when someone has an issue with you:**

- Go to the person you harmed or offended. Do not make them come to you.
- Hear the other person out completely and consider what they say before responding.
- Search your heart and the Lord to discover the truth in the situation.
- Offer an honest apology and repent of any wrongdoing.
- Ask for their forgiveness and ask the Lord to forgive you as well.
- Abide by their wishes regarding how to move forward in the relationship. Do not force forgiveness or push for relationship if they, or you, are reluctant.
- Once you did all you can do, leave the rest in God's hands.

*So if you are offering your gift at the altar and there <u>remember that your brother has something against you, leave your gift there before the altar and go</u>. First be reconciled to your brother, and then come and offer your gift.*
*(Matthew 5:23 – 24)*

## When the Issue Is with Someone Who Hurt You

"If possible, so far as it depends on you, live peaceably with all" (Romans 12:18). This verse still applies when you are harmed. Examine your heart to see how you may have wronged the other person. In most conflicts, **both people** make mistakes. If needed, start the conversation with an apology to set a tone for reconciliation, but **keep your apology genuine** and do not use it to introduce blame.

- A poor apology would be, "I am sorry I hung up on you, but you are so unreasonable."

- A better apology would be, "I am sorry, I hung up on you. I did not handle my emotions well. I am sorry I hurt your feelings."

**Some things to remember when handling an offense:**

➢ **Understand the situation.** Journal about the situation to get it clear in your mind.

- o What was the exact nature of the wrong against me?
- o What was my part in it? How do I feel? How did I respond?
- o What is the perspective of the others involved? How might they feel? What emotions led each person's response?
- o What was the impact on my life? What did the person's actions threaten?
- o What is God's truth? Am I believing the report of the enemy?

➢ **Get right with God.**

- o Did I handle the situation biblically? Where do I need to repent?
- o Is there an error or character defect in myself that I saw reflected in the other person, or that influenced my response?
- o Confess your wrongs to God and seek His forgiveness. Stand ready to forgive the other person for their wrongs to you, regardless of the conflict's outcome.

➢ **See the offender through the loving eyes of God.**

- o Remember God's grace and mercy in your life. Have compassion for your offender.
- o Remember it is God's nature to restore the offender, just as He wants to restore you.
- o Ask the Lord to guide you to reconciliation. The purpose of conflict is to restore wholeness in the relationship, **not to prove that you are right**.

➢ **Prepare yourself for conflict.**

- o Prepare your heart to seek the best for both the offender and you in love.
- o Prepare your ears to listen to their side.
- o Prepare your eyes to see the other person's perspective.
- o Prepare your hands to extend grace, mercy, and truth.
- o Prepare your feet to walk on the path of peace, searching for reconciliation.
- o Prepare your mouth to give answers seasoned with meekness, humility, and respect.

➢ **Confront the one who hurt you.**

  o This is a two-way conversation, and the other's feelings and thoughts may differ from yours. Even though you were wronged, it is important to show the offender respect.

  o Tell the other how you were wrong and ask for forgiveness.

  o Seek clarification, and prepare questions you can ask. This will help you stay on track and focus on finding the truth rather than allowing your emotions to guide the discussion.

  o Tell the offender only what you need him to know about how his actions affected you. Do not bring up past, **resolved** offenses to prove your point.

  o Be gentle and consider their feelings while being firm and straightforward.

  o Use non-threatening communication, such as "I" statements. ("I think," "I feel," "I hope," etc.)

  o Discuss what each person needs to resolve the matter.

➢ **Restoration**

  o If the person listens to you and you both believe the matter is resolved, let the offender know you forgive them and do not continue rehashing the offense.

  o Pray with them and be ready to help the offender overcome his or her transgression.

## When the Offender Does Not Listen

What do you do when you try your best to resolve a matter, but the offender refuses to listen?

> *__If your brother sins against you, go and tell him his fault__, between you and him alone. If he listens to you, you have gained your brother. But if he does not listen, take one or two others along with you, that every charge may be established by the evidence of two or three witnesses. If he refuses to listen to them, tell it to the church. And if he refuses to listen even to the church, let him be to you as a Gentile and a tax collector.*
> *(Matthew 18:15 – 17)*

**Take one or two others to bear witness**

After attempting resolution with the person one on one, it is okay to take others with you to confront the problem. The implication in this verse in Matthew 18 is **to bring objective people** whose goals are **restoration**, who seek the best interests of both parties, listen with impartiality, and are willing to extend grace and mercy. This verse is not an excuse to **gather allies** that will gang up on the offender and fight your point.

**Take it before the church**

This is how you handle conflict **with believers**. Obviously, it is not appropriate to drag a non-believer before your church elders to show how they are wrong. How can you hold a non-believer to Christian standards? When an issue with a non-believer cannot be resolved, leave it in the Lord's hands and distance yourself to prevent future harm.

**Treat the offender like a Gentile**

After every attempt has failed and the individual is clearly unrepentant, "let him be to you as a Gentile or tax collector." Paul shows us what this means in his letters to the churches. The one treated as a "Gentile or a tax collector" is separated from the body of believers, treated like a non-believer, and **put on a path toward repentance for his salvation**. This is meant to be done in love; it is not an excuse to shun him or be cruel. You do not "ghost" the offender or treat him like a leper. Make the problem clear and continue to love and pray for him. The separation puts him in the Lord's hands and protects other believers from his sin. God draws the offender in to deal with his heart.

> *If anyone does not obey what we say in this letter, take note of that person, and have nothing to do with him, that he may be ashamed. Do not regard him as an enemy, but warn him as a brother. (2 Thessalonians 3:15)*

> *You are to deliver this man to Satan for the destruction of the flesh, so that his spirit may be saved in the day of the Lord. (1 Corinthians 5:5)*

**Restoring the offender**

When the offender realizes his wrongs and chooses change, **be quick to restore him**. If the offender's **repentance is genuine**, even if he repeats past mistakes, he will correct them. **He should return to open and loving arms, comfort, forgiveness, rejoicing, and a fresh start.** Reaffirm your love for him. Do not hold his past wrongs against him but give him the opportunity to earn your trust again.

> *For such a one, this punishment by the majority is enough, so you should rather turn to forgive and comfort him, or he may be overwhelmed by excessive sorrow.  So I beg you to reaffirm your love for him. (2 Corinthians 2:6 – 8)*

> *As it is, I rejoice, not because you were grieved, but because you were grieved into repenting. For you felt a godly grief, so that you suffered no loss through us. For godly grief produces a repentance that leads to salvation without regret, whereas worldly grief produces death. (2 Corinthians 7:9 – 10)*

## Questions to Ponder

48.9)   What did you learn you should do differently when a conflict arises?

48.10) Is there a current situation to which you can apply this lesson? Explain.

48.11) Explain the difference between handling conflict with a believer and handling conflict with a non-believer.

48.12) Have you restored someone as described in this lesson? What was the result?

# Lesson 49 — Communication

**The way we communicate will always reflect either Christ or the world.** It is difficult to communicate in God's love when our emotions are out of control. Preconceived ideas about a person can influence the way we communicate with them. People often hear what they expect, rather than the actual words spoken. **The key to effective communication is for each person to honor the other in the way they listen and the words they speak.**

## Effective Listening

❖ **Actively Listen** – Active listening honors the one who is speaking. Instead of planning your reply, give your full focus to comprehending the message the other is trying to convey. It is easy to listen from your perspective and assume a person thinks like you. Ask questions to discover the point that **the speaker** wants you to understand. Give the speaker your full attention and maintain eye contact (but do not stare—that is creepy).

> *Know this, my beloved brothers: let every person be quick to hear,*
> *slow to speak, slow to anger. (James 1:19)*

❖ **Avoid Interrupting** – This is easier said than done, especially when you are a quick thinker, or someone is long-winded. Allow the speaker full expression of his or her thought. The person will feel heard, and you will gain a clearer understanding of their message. Sometimes it helps to jot down notes as a reminder of what they said to address it later, allowing your full focus to stay on the one speaking.

> *A fool takes no pleasure in understanding, but only in expressing his opinion.*
> *(Proverbs 18:2)*

> *If one gives an answer before he hears, it is his folly and shame.*
> *(Proverbs 18:13)*

❖ **Avoid Distraction** – Do not allow pets, children, or other environmental factors to draw your attention away from the speaker. If possible, turn off your phone or silence the notifications.

> *For everything there is a season, and a time for every matter under heaven.*
> *(Ecclesiastes 3:1)*

❖ **Keep an Open Mind** – Do not look for what is wrong in another's words, but listen from his perspective. Listen with impartiality. You may learn something new, or it may alert you to a wrong understanding. Wait for the speaker to finish before deciding whether you agree or disagree.

> *The heart of the righteous ponders how to answer, but the mouth of the*
> *wicked pours out evil things. (Proverbs 15:28)*

## Effective Speaking

- ❖ **Speak Truth in Love** – Make sure your words are honest. In love, speak your genuine thoughts and feelings, even if you know the person will disagree with you. Do not avoid speaking truth to spare someone's feelings but speak with gentleness and compassion when sharing a hard truth. Do not make up stories, exaggerate, or leave out important details. If you cannot speak truth, it is best to say nothing.

  *Rather, speaking the truth in love, we are to grow up in every way
  into him who is the head, into Christ. (Ephesians 4:15)*

  *Better is open rebuke than hidden love. Faithful are the wounds of a friend;
  profuse are the kisses of an enemy. (Proverbs 27:5 – 6)*

- ❖ **Be Direct** – Do not talk around an issue to avoid answering a question, hoping a person will "read between the lines." Do not give a disingenuous answer. **Being misunderstood contradicts the purpose of communication.** Get straight to the point and give full, clear descriptions, details, and examples to communicate an unmistakable message to the listener.

  *The heart of the wise makes his speech judicious and adds persuasiveness to his lips.
  (Proverbs 16:23)*

- ❖ **Use Kind Words** – Honor other people with your words, remembering that unkind words can hurt. Your tongue holds the power of life and death. Before you speak, think about how your words may sound to another. Avoid rejection, avoidance, scorn, sarcasm, ridicule, threats, accusing, or blaming. These are cruel, abusive, and ineffective in communication.

  *Let your speech always be gracious, seasoned with salt, so that you may
  know how you ought to answer each person. (Colossians 4:6)*

  *A gentle tongue is a tree of life, but perverseness in it breaks the spirit. (Proverbs 15:4)*

  *There is one whose rash words are like sword thrusts, but the tongue of the wise brings healing.
  (Proverbs 12:18)*

  *Whoever belittles his neighbor lacks sense, but a man of understanding remains silent.
  (Proverbs 11:12)*

- ❖ **Use "I" Statements** – Use "I" statements every time you are sad, angry, defensive, or need to confront another person about an issue. It is far more effective to focus your speech on yourself than on another. When the word "you" is used to address a problem, it puts the listener on the defensive. No one wants to hear how they are wrong, but they are more open to hearing you say "I think" or "I feel." Instead of saying, "You left dirty dishes in the sink again," say, "I am upset that the dishes were not done." Or, instead of saying, "Why don't you fix this?" say, "It would help me to know your plans about this." Use "I" statements to express thoughts, feelings, concerns, or to share how a behavior affects you. Then state what you need to happen.

*A soft answer turns away wrath, but a harsh word stirs up anger. (Proverbs 15:1)*

*To speak evil of no one, to avoid quarreling, to be gentle, and to show perfect courtesy toward all people. (Titus 3:2)*

## Body Language

❖ **Your Body Speaks Louder Than Your Words.** Keep open body language as you engage in communication. Assume a listening position, unguarded and engaged. Your face will give you away if you are disingenuous. If your expressions are interested and reflect the other's feelings, the person will trust your words are genuine. **Your body will speak your language** if you are open and honest.

*A worthless person, a wicked man, goes about with crooked speech, winks with his eyes, signals with his feet, points with his finger, with perverted heart devises evil, continually sowing discord. (Proverbs 6:12 – 14)*

*But I discipline my body and keep it under control, lest after preaching to others I myself should be disqualified. (1 Corinthians 9:27)*

### Questions to Ponder

49.1) Are your listening skills effective? Where can you improve?

49.2) How can you become more attentive while listening? What distracts you from listening?

49.3) Do you interrupt? Are you considering your response while another is talking?

49.4) How open are you to hearing another person's perspective?

49.5) Are your speaking skills effective? Where can you improve?

49.6) How honest is your communication? Do you say what others expect or want to hear? Do you exaggerate or leave out details?

49.7) Is your communication direct and to the point, or do you try to get your message across without saying what is truly on your mind?

49.8) Do you use many details and examples to make sure your messages are clear?

49.9) Are you thoughtful? How often do you use sarcasm, ridicule, threats, accusations, or blame, to respond to another's questions or comments? Do you ignore them?

## Effective Communication

Effective communication may be difficult when you or another have a vested interest in the conversation's outcome. **Be intentional about how you communicate.** The following tips can help:

❖ **Observe the Conversation** – Use your emotions to teach you; do not allow them to control you. Prepare your mind to observe the conversation and actions of others without absorbing their negativity. Let their words roll off you. When you focus your mind on observing, it is more difficult to absorb the other person's words as a personal attack.

> *Do not take to heart all the things that people say, lest you hear your servant cursing you.*
> *Your heart knows that many times you yourself have cursed others.*
> *(Ecclesiastes 7:21 – 22)*

❖ **Do not Become Vexed** – Vexation is when we feel worried, annoyed, or frustrated. One of the greatest traps laid by the enemy is to use other people to push our buttons. Once we lose patience and show annoyance or irritation, we lose the conversation. There is an old saying that you catch more flies with honey than with vinegar. You may not want to catch flies, but this old saying still rings true. When your responses become grumpy or bitter people stop listening. On the other hand, it is impossible to escalate a conflict with someone who always replies sweetly and refuses to be baited into a heated quarrel. Gentle kindness and patience will serve you well.  Do not become discouraged when you mess up. Strong emotions make it difficult to respond in love. Keep trying. It will get easier.

> *The vexation of a fool is known at once, but the prudent ignores an insult. (Proverbs 12:16)*

> *With patience a ruler may be persuaded, and a soft tongue will break a bone. (Proverbs 25:15)*

❖ **Be Discerning** – Always seek the Lord's wisdom when communicating with another. Listen for subtle manipulations and falsehoods but respond with kindness. Your integrity is more important than making sure they understand your emotional state. Redirect conversation back to the truth. Use wisdom when deciding what you share and how you speak.

> *The wise of heart is called discerning, and sweetness of speech increases persuasiveness.*
> *(Proverbs 16:21)*

❖ **Respond, Don't React** – Respond to the situation; do not react to it. We **react** in emotion; we plan **responses**. Reactions further turmoil while responses will guide you through the problem. Once your handling of a situation becomes unreasonable, intense emotions overshadow everything you say. Plan a calm, reasoned response.

> *Whoever is slow to anger has great understanding, but he who has a hasty temper exalts folly.*
> *(Proverbs 14:29)*

## Planned Communication

When approaching a conflict or difficult conversation, you need a good grasp on what you are thinking and why. When something causes a powerful emotion, do not storm out to confront the person. Instead, make a plan to communicate. Having a plan makes a favorable outcome more likely.

**Before communicating**

- ❖ **Allow Plenty of Time** – Plan to engage in a serious conversation when neither party feels stress and there is plenty of time available. Do not force or rush a conversation.

- ❖ **Identify Your Emotions and Their Causes** – Know what you feel and why you feel it. Often, the easiest answer is not the only answer. Repeat the question "Why else do I feel this way?" until you can no longer answer. This helps you see a bigger picture of the situation and may help you determine an appropriate course of action.

  - ○ **Example:** I feel angry about_____. I also feel angry about _____. I also feel angry about_____. (Repeat for all emotions: fear, sadness, etc.)

- ❖ **Review the Elements of Effective Speaking and Listening in This Lesson** – It takes a lot of practice to learn alternative methods of communication. Practice prepares you for more challenging conversations.

**During communication**

- ❖ **Encourage Successful Communication** – You may have excellent communication skills, but that does not mean that the one you are conversing with does. You can, however, direct the conversation to improve communication.

- ❖ **Do Not Overwhelm the Listener** – State clear and precise points using "I" statements. Only offer **one point on one issue** at a time. If you rattle off twenty points at once, it is impossible for the listener to address them all. When confronted with many issues, people often focus on the one they are most comfortable addressing. If you are a listener in this scenario, ask the speaker to return to their first point and deal with issues one by one. They will probably return to the point they consider most important to address.

- ❖ **Ask the Listener to Repeat Your Point** – Many times, conversations go wrong because the listener is not actively listening. Having the listener repeat what you said is a simple way to make sure they clearly understood you.

  - ○ **Example:** "Can you tell me what I said in your own words, so I know you understand me?"

- ❖ **Move on to the Next Point** – After you are certain the other person understands you, move on to the next point. Do not engage in a discussion on each point until you finish speaking, and do not allow the conversation to veer toward a new issue. Ask the listener to hear you out before responding. You may suggest they take notes on something they wish to address after you finish. If they refuse to hear you out, end the conversation until they are ready to listen.

- ❖ **Hear the Other Side** – After you have finished expressing every point, give the listener the same opportunity to respond. Ask them also to state one point at a time and repeat each point back to them: "I heard you say that_____." **Show them the same respect you demand for yourself.** Do not interrupt or cut them off, and make sure you comprehend their message.

**After communicating**

- ❖ **Make Your Decision** – Once everyone has expressed their thoughts and feelings, end the conversation: "I will consider/pray about what you said." Refuse to **offer or hint** to an answer until you have an opportunity to consider it. Do not allow yourself to be rushed. **Give answers like**, "I understand what you are saying" or "I understand how you feel". **Do not give answers like**, "You may be right" or "Maybe later" or "I think I can _____." These kinds of answers create an opening to be manipulated into making a snap decision. Only give an answer after reflecting and praying about it away from the conversation.

- ❖ **Tell the Other Person Your Decision** – Once you decide about the conversation, tell the other person the truth. Discuss the points on which you agree **and** disagree with them. If the conversation led to a choice, tell them your decision.

## A Model to Approach a Difficult Conversation

Use the following model to start a tough conversation. This model will help you approach the person in a loving and non-threatening way.

- ❖ **I know/believe that you _____.** Explain your understanding of the other person's perspective—what you believe they expect, feel, think, or are doing, and why. This helps assure the person of your effort to understand them. It may also clarify the cause of a misunderstanding from the start.

- ❖ **I have been trying to_____.** What are you doing to abide by their wishes, respect their feelings, or correct the situation?

- ❖ **I feel_____when _____.** What is the issue you want to discuss?

- ❖ **I would like to see_____.** How do you see the issue resolving?

*I tell you, on the day of judgment people will give account for every careless word they speak. For by your words you will be justified, and by your words you will be condemned. (Matthew 12:36 – 37)*

*Set a guard, O Lord, over my mouth; keep watch over the door of my lips! (Psalm 141:3)*

*Even a fool who keeps silent is considered wise; when he closes his lips, he is deemed intelligent. (Proverbs 17:28)*

## Questions to Ponder

49.10) Practice effective listening and effective speaking this week. Write about three times you used these skills and the result of using them.

49.11) Use the planned communication skills and model to have a difficult conversation. When it is finished, reflect: What was the result? Did you find it easy to use?

49.12) Ask your coach to practice these techniques with you.

# Chapter Nineteen

## Keep Growing
## & Move

# Lesson 50 — Make Your Recovery Grow

Just when you think you know God, He reveals more. If you spent your lifetime studying God's Word, you would never come close to understanding all God's attributes.

*If anyone imagines that he knows something, he does not yet know as he ought to know.*
*(1 Corinthians 8:2)*

There is always a deeper level of relationship and spiritual growth to attain. Do not think you have arrived. The Lord continues to raise you from one level of glory to the next. It only gets better! **Here, your purpose is found in the journey, not the destination.** God sealed the destination the day you gave your life over to Christ. Hold fast to the truths you know but continue to press on to greater things that lie ahead. In this life, it is the journey that matters.

*Not that I have already obtained it [this goal of being Christlike] or have already been*
*made perfect, but I actively press on so that I may take hold of that [perfection] for*
*which Christ Jesus took hold of me and made me His own. Brothers and sisters, I do*
*not consider that I have made it my own yet; but one thing I do: forgetting what lies*
*behind and reaching forward to what lies ahead, I press on toward the goal to win*
*the [heavenly] prize of the upward call of God in Christ Jesus. All of us who are mature*
*[pursuing spiritual perfection] should have this attitude. And if in any respect you*
*have a different attitude, that too God will make clear to you. Only let us stay true to*
*what we have already attained. (Philippians 3:12-16 (AMP))*

*And we all, with unveiled face, beholding the glory of the Lord, are being transformed*
*into the same image from one degree of glory to another. For this comes from the*
*Lord who is the Spirit. (2 Corinthians 3:18)*

The rest of your *Rebuilt* lessons will focus on ways to maintain the progress you have made, deal with additional issues as they arise, build healthy habits, and continue to grow ever closer to the Lord. Moving forward requires stepping into a new level of relationship with the Lord to allow His work to grow deeper in your heart.

## Questions to Ponder

50.1) Is there anything stopping you from giving your all to Christ? Explain.

50.2) What do you think is the difference between living for Christ and abiding in Him?

50.3) What would your life look like if you began living from Him?

56

## Stop Living for Christ, and Begin Living from Him

If you were asked how you live for Christ, what would you say? You read your Bible, serve your neighbors, serve your church? Are you a prayer warrior? These are important activities for a believer, but if you are not abiding in Christ; they are mere works of your flesh.

Jesus requires more; He requires that we abide in Him. To abide is to remain or continue in Him, to live or dwell in Him. Scripture says we are to lose our lives to save them. Our lives do not belong to us; rather, God bought us for a price. Do you understand the depth of what this means? **The cost of following Christ is giving up your life and living from His.**

*For although there may be so-called gods in heaven or on earth—as indeed there are many "gods" and many "lords"— yet for us there is one God, the Father, <u>from whom are all things and for whom we exist</u>, and one Lord, Jesus Christ, through <u>whom are all things and through whom we exist</u>. (1 Corinthians 8:5 – 6)*

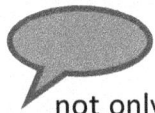

"Therefore, you must put Him first and then let everything flow from that. Let everything begin with Him and flow forth from Him. That's the secret of life. To not only live for Him, but to live your life from Him, to live from His living, to move from His moving, to act from His actions, to feel from His heart, to be from His being, and to become who you are from who He is ... I am."

Jonathan Cahn, *The Book of Mysteries* (Lake Mary, FL: Frontline, 2016). Used with permission.

God created you unique. His command to give up your life does not suggest giving up the specific traits that make you, <u>you</u>. Instead, it means to submit all of who you are to Christ's will and authority. When you are "all in," you can claim with Paul, "It is no longer I who live but Christ in me" (Galatians 2:20). This is the place where you stop living from your flesh.

The name of God is literally "I AM." His very breath formed everything; all that exists came from his being. **He is our source, which gives us life and sustains us.** Without Christ we are a dying mound of flesh trying to find life in artificial sources, such as our job, friends, success, wealth, family, and even our morals. These are false gods and idols that **give us a false sense of living** but cannot truly give us abundant life.

*I have been crucified with Christ. It is no longer I who live, but Christ who lives in me. And the life I now live in the flesh I live by faith in the Son of God, who loved me and gave himself for me. (Galatians 2:20)*

Our source must change. **When the world is our source, we live from our need, but when God is our source, we live from Christ's abundance.** Let the essence of who you are, your thoughts, actions, and desires, flow from Him. Allow your "I am" to flow from the "I AM."

To abide in Christ and allow him to abide in you is, in effect, **becoming one with God**. The old corrupt nature no longer has room to exist. As you rise to life in Christ, every surrendered part of you takes on His likeness. Your life becomes Jesus' hands and feet to a lost world. Every word you speak and every thought in your mind is birthed by His wisdom, and He guides each step of your feet.

You would not intentionally remove a limb, pluck out an eyeball, or cut out a healthy organ. **God is part of you, and you are part of Him.** Trying to move without Him would be little different from trying to run a marathon without your legs. Living life **for** God instead of **from** Him is like running a race with artificial limbs. A prosthetic limb can help you get your life back after a devastating injury, but you will never be fully connected to it.

Our sin caused a handicap, which prevents us from living the way God first designed us to live. **In our flesh, we seek artificial gods** to fill this missing part of us. As **believers, we may rely on our religious works** and our understanding, yet we can only become whole by **becoming one with God. He is the missing piece** of our being, which makes us complete.

*But he who is joined to the Lord becomes one spirit with him. (1 Corinthians 6:17)*

*If then you have been raised with Christ, seek the things that are above, where Christ is, seated at the right hand of God. Set your minds on things that are above, not on things that are on earth. For you have died, and your life is hidden with Christ in God. When Christ who is your life appears, then you also will appear with him in glory. (Colossians 3:1 – 4)*

> ## Questions to Ponder
>
> 50.4) Considering what you have just read, how would you define living *from* Christ?
>
> 50.5) How will this look in your life?

## Put on the Blinders!

If you have ever witnessed a crime or accident, you know each person's story is different. This does not mean that one person is lying, and another is speaking truth. It is a matter of perspective. Each witness has a distinct vantage point, and as a result, each narrative of the same event varies. None of the witnesses see the complete picture; they can only speak to what each personally saw. Their testimonies are like puzzle pieces. The investigator attempts to fit all the pieces together to form a big picture and discern the truth.

**Your eyes are your witnesses**, taking in information about current circumstances. **Your mind is the investigator**, making assumptions based on what your eyes perceive, but these are often flawed assumptions. Your witnesses only see from the narrow perspective that revolves around you, filtered through desires, preconceived ideas, worldview, and experiences. **God, however, sees the big picture we cannot comprehend.** He sees details of the heart, which no person can witness. Abiding in Christ allows **a new understanding** from God's perspective, **with healthy eyes** focused on the eternal.

*That the God of our Lord Jesus Christ, the Father of glory, may give you the Spirit of wisdom and of revelation in the knowledge of him, having the eyes of your hearts enlightened, that you may know what is the hope to which he has called you, what are the riches of his glorious inheritance in the saints. (Ephesians 1:17 – 18)*

*The eye is the lamp of the body. So, if your eye is healthy, your whole body will be full of light. (Matthew 6:22)*

## Discover a God Perspective

The Lord can open the eyes of your heart to new revelation and understanding. It is far easier to seek His truth in times devoted to worship, prayer, and study. When finances, people, and situations become overwhelming, or your desires in life conflict with God's, focusing on the eternal can seem like an impossible task.

**To walk in God's truth, put blinders on your natural eyes and see with God's perspective**. This is something many believers spend their lives unable to grasp because we function in a natural world. Those who grasp it, like the first believers, live abundant lives, walking with God in boldness, confidence, and contentment.

**Use the following suggestions to live life with the mind of Christ:**

❖ **Stop Trying to Make God Fit Your Life** – Ask to come into the Lord's presence **to walk with Him** through **His** day. Do not try to make God **or His word** fit your life; instead, make your life fit with Scripture and God's plan. Your relationship with the Lord comes first. Do not worry about what others do; focus on what **you** are doing. When He leads your days, He shows you how to live rightly, who to pray for, and who needs help.

❖ **Do Not Stop Moving** –The law of inertia in physics states that something in motion or rest will stay in motion or rest until acted upon by an outside force. This principle can be applied to your relationship with God. Once you start moving with God, you will continue moving with Him unless an outside force stops you. **Distractions become the force that stops your forward movement with God.** When you are living **for** Christ, any crisis, financial burden, political issue, person, or distraction of the world can take your mind off Him. When your life flows **from** His, directed by His leading, the mundane and difficult tasks of life will not draw you away but bring you closer to Him. Are you giving your attention to worthy things, or are you distracted?

❖ **Rest in God, Not in the World** –It is easy to turn your attention off the Lord to just "live your life." **To be one with God means we can't take a break from Him.** Remember, He bought you for a price; it is not **your** life you are living, but His. He is part of you, and you are part of Him. To claim that you require a break from God is like demanding a break from your right arm.

❖ **How You Rest Matters** –We often confuse entertainment with rest. Have you ever come home from vacation exhausted? Your break **left you entertained, but not rested**. To rest in the Lord, is taking a break from life's burdens to focus your attention on Jesus. True rest is **not fulfilling a litany of religious duties, but** devoting time to **simply enjoy God**, spending intimate time with Him alone, in His creation, or in fellowship with His people. Play is important too, but not at the expense of resting in the Lord. His rest keeps you moving forward. Mind-numbing pursuits or worldly entertainment are not rest but distractions.

❖ **Do Not Grow Weary of Doing God's Work** – You know you have taken back the control you once gave the Lord when you neglect your walk with Christ. Neglecting prayer, study, or worship is a clue that your rest is laziness. You will remain idle until an **outside force**, such as a trial or crisis, brings you back to the feet of the Lord.

❖ **Stop Taking God for Granted; Take Evil for Granted** – We live in a fallen world, and bad things happen. Evil exists. Take this truth for granted. The expectation that bad things happen focuses our eyes on the Lord's blessings, fixing our thoughts on God and strengthening our faith. When we take God and his goodness for granted, every trial and evil grabs our attention. Troubles seem bigger, and doubt creeps in. We may wonder, "Where is God?" or "Why hasn't God acted?" and our faith wavers.

❖ **Remember, Everything Works for Good** – Our minds create a concept of good and bad to determine how we view a situation. This perspective is often founded on what we like or dislike. This is a worldly perspective. When we have the mind of Christ, we can experience joy in our trials because they work for our perfection and completion. God makes "bad" circumstances benefit us, and He blesses us with "good" gifts. When you encounter hardships, focus on the Lord and how He is using the situation to finish His work in you.

## Today Starts a New Journey

Let today begin a new journey with the Lord, one that takes you into a deeper relationship, where you stop living for Christ and start living from Him. No longer think of or address the Lord as if He is separate from you. Live as one entity, working for an eternal purpose greater than this world. This is living in truth. Today, as you continue your journey, **you have a choice**. Do you stay where you are, or jump "all in" with Christ?

---

**We exist *for* God, but our existence flows *from* Him.
We live from Him and through Him.**

❖ It is not about applying the word to your life but living your life from His word.
❖ It is not making scripture fit your life; it is making your life fit the scripture.
❖ It is not about inviting Him to walk with you through your day, it is about asking to come into His presence and walk with Him through His day.

---

Questions to Ponder

50.6)   What is the main understanding you have taken away from this lesson?

50.7)   How will you apply a new perspective as you move forward with God?

50.8)   How can you change the way you enter God's presence each day?

50.9)   Are you setting your attention on activities that do not benefit God's purpose?

50.10)  Have you made a choice to be "all in" with God? If not, why not?

50.11)  How have you taken God for granted?

50.12)  How can you take evil for granted?

# Lesson 51 — Preventing Relapse

Satan's strongholds have fallen and now your only stronghold is the Lord. The enemy's arrows bounce off the shield of your faith. Your adversary once fought hard to keep you away from God. He lost that battle, yet he does not lose graciously. His attacks will continue, but now **his goals have changed**. How do you walk through life without falling into former detrimental thoughts and behaviors?

**It is important for you to be aware of the enemy's new strategy. He wants to**

- **Make you ineffective** for God's Kingdom

- **Tempt you back** into old strongholds

- **Destroy your confidence** in an area God has gifted you

Paul was no stranger to spiritual warfare. He understood that **we have three enemies fighting against us** as we live out a spiritual life with Christ:

- We wrestle spiritual **powers and principalities** of darkness and evil

- We struggle against the **world** (people and systems against God), which hates God and His people

- We battle our own **flesh**

*For we do not wrestle against flesh and blood, but against the rulers, against the authorities, against the cosmic powers over this present darkness, against the spiritual forces of evil in the heavenly places. (Ephesians 6:12)*

Obvious demonic or "supernatural" activity may come about because you have opened a door through occult activity or influences, witchcraft, or other agreement held with the devil. You must break your agreement with the enemy and come into agreement with God so you can rebuke the devil in Jesus' name. This may require prayer and fasting. If you feel you need help with demonic attacks or oppression, consult with your *Rebuilt* coach.

Some people understand "spiritual powers and principalities" as only referring to demonic activity, but often **spiritual authorities are subtle, disguising their attacks in what appears good or right in our eyes**. They ally with our flesh and the world to prevent us from pursuing our calling and advancing the Kingdom of God.

Our spiritual enemy attacks our mind, using our flesh to cause thoughts of rejection, loss, desire, anger, or fear. His purpose is to tempt us away from Christ and our calling and cause bouts of depression, temptation, or anxiety. **However, we do not need the devil to sin or tempt us. Our own sin nature may draw us away if we do not keep it in check** by walking with the Holy Spirit. Spiritual enemies may use people, even well-meaning people, to carry out their assignments. **It is vital that you refuse to be a slave to the opinions of man**, testing everything by the Word of God and seeking His confirmation. Rebuke thoughts and ideas contrary to truth. When we are walking with God, the enemy has no power, and our spirit testifies to the truth. We need not worry.

> *But I say, walk by the Spirit, and you will not gratify the desires of the flesh. For the desires of the flesh are against the Spirit, and the desires of the Spirit are against the flesh, for these are opposed to each other, to keep you from doing the things you want to do. (Galatians 5:16 – 17)*

Paul understood how to walk with the Lord without falling into these traps. He encouraged believers to follow his example, and the example of those who walk as he did with the Lord.

> *Brothers, join in imitating me, and keep your eyes on those who walk according to the example you have in us. (Philippians 3:17)*

There are several key things we can learn from Paul's example. In Philippians 3, Paul defines a pattern for life that we should walk in as believers. As we dig into this chapter, we discover this pattern helps us **avoid relapse and walk in freedom** with God.

## 1. Choose Your Friends Wisely

> ***Look out for the dogs, look out for the evildoers, look out for those who mutilate the flesh. (Philippians 3:2)***

Paul tells us to be careful whom we choose to associate with. It matters. As you continue with life after *Rebuilt*, it may be easy to forget what you have learned. You may feel temptation to restore toxic relationships because you assume you can handle them now. The truth is bad company corrupts; at best it may lead your mind away from the Lord. It is vital to your recovery and future journey with the Lord to make careful decisions regarding the people and influences you allow in your life.

*Rebuilt* has taught you a great deal about avoiding the influence, control, and manipulation of toxic people, **yet anyone can be detrimental to you if you become a slave to their opinions**. When you desire the approval of any person more than God's approval, even those you love, Scripture says you are undeserving of God. The desire for acceptance moves you to compromise your values, your boldness, and your confidence in the Lord, and it **limits you to another person's will**. Any person's opinion that holds more weight than the Lord's will become the "dogs" in the above verse that stop you from reaching your full potential in God. **You do not need to earn the approval of others or fear offending them by your beliefs and opinions.** Find people who accept you and sharpen you without judgment and condemnation; find people "equally yoked."

> *Whoever loves father or mother more than me is not worthy of me, and whoever loves son or daughter more than me is not worthy of me. (Matthew 10:37)*

> *For am I now seeking the approval of man, or of God? Or am I trying to please man? If I were still trying to please man, I would not be a servant of Christ. (Galatians 1:10)*

*And he said to them, "You are those who justify yourselves before men, but God knows your hearts. For what is exalted among men is an abomination in the sight of God." (Luke 16:15)*

<u>Questions to Ponder</u>

51.1) Whom do you value time with more than time with God?

51.2) Whose opinions do you value over God's?

51.3) What ways do you care about people's opinions?

51.4) Do you compromise your behavior to gain approval or your words to please or not offend another?

51.5) Do you fear people thinking you are wrong? Do you often argue your opinions?

## 2. Be Confident

*For we are the circumcision, who worship by the Spirit of God and glory in Christ Jesus and <u>put no confidence in the flesh</u>. (Philippians 3:3)*

Of course, as believers we must worship God, giving glory to Jesus, but this verse speaks to more than whom we worship. **Where we place our confidence matters**.

Place your confidence **in your relationship and identity in Christ, in your ability to hear His voice, and in His sovereignty over the outcome of any situation.** You can be confident because it is not your ability you rely on, but God's. Lack of confidence in God gives the enemy a foothold to condemn, shame, frighten, or deceive you. If your confidence is in God and His truth about you, doubt will not become a stumbling block.

Confidence also produces an excitement and boldness for Christ. Your confidence is your witness. Can you imagine telling someone about your love for Christ without confidence in who He is and in your testimony? Who would believe you?

As you continue to walk with the Lord, the enemy may seek to defeat you with condemnation, claiming you are not enough or a failure. He may turn your attention from God's truth back to the opinions of man, tempting you to fear rejection or ridicule. He plays on fears of loss. He speaks doubt, causing you to wonder if the Lord left or is punishing you because you did not "perform" well enough for Him. Remember, all these ideas are lies from hell.

God's mercy is new each morning. **Failure does not equal the end, but an opportunity for growth.** Which is more valuable and truer, God's or man's opinion? You are loved. God knows what you go through. **Trials are a mere steppingstone to a new level of glory** in Christ. Have confidence, because with God your only limits are His convictions; your **possibilities** are limitless!

When doubt and insecurity plague your mind, remember this truth:
The question is not if you are able, but rather if God can make you able.
And He can!

**Confidence is not pride**

**Beware of pride.** The enemy feeds on pride to make you ineffective for the Kingdom. Our confidence must be in God, not the flesh. Do not forget that Christ is the source of your victory and healing. It is tempting to think, "I've got this!" but you have nothing without Him. Do not forsake trusting in God for trusting in your own understanding or ability. Your assurance in the outcome of a situation comes from your confidence in God.

**Paul continues in verses 4 – 6** to state why he has more than enough reason to be confident. In his flesh, he was righteous under the law, blameless, from the tribe of Benjamin, a zealous Pharisee. The religious world considered him a successful, prominent man, yet he chose confidence not in himself, but in Christ Jesus. **We must do the same.**

No matter how smart or educated we are, or how much scriptural knowledge we possess, our faith belongs in God, not ourselves. We can do good works and give excellent gifts, but without God in us, all our works are like filthy rags. Stay confident in your identity and ability **in Christ**, because your God makes you able to do amazing things.

> *We have all become like one who is unclean, and <u>all our righteous deeds are like a polluted garment</u>. We all fade like a leaf, and our iniquities, like the wind, take us away.* *(Isaiah 64:6)*

## Questions to Ponder

51.6) List evidence of your identity in Christ to revisit when your confidence fails. List times you heard the Lord's voice, how He has used you, and times He intervened in situations. List times that God showed up when you messed up.

51.7) Are you enough, as you are, for God? Why or why not?

51.8) How confident are you that you can do "all things through Christ"?

51.9) How do you still struggle with pride?

51.10) In what circumstances do you currently attempt to solve or understand situations in your own power or wisdom?

## 3. Gratitude and Reflection

> *But whatever gain I had, I counted as loss for the sake of Christ. Indeed, I count everything as loss because of the surpassing worth of knowing Christ Jesus my Lord. For his sake I have suffered the loss of all things and count them as rubbish, in order that I may gain Christ, and be found in him, not having a righteousness of my own that comes from the law, but that which comes through faith in Christ, the righteousness from God that depends on faith.*
> *(Philippians 3:7 – 9)*

After describing his prior success and notable stature, Paul reflects on what he once had, stating it was all loss, garbage, rubbish. **Nothing was worth more than what he gained through relationship with Christ.** Paul experienced shipwreck and isolation, torment, torture, imprisonment, and became a martyr for his beliefs, yet he considered his life to be more fulfilling and of higher value with Christ than without Him.

As you continue walking with the Lord, take time to remember everything have gained. Your journals serve as an altar of remembrance to God's miracles in you. Review them as a reminder of how far the Lord has brought you. **Your journey is the evidence you need** to trust God's work and provision in your life when trials shake your hope and faith.

You may think you can never forget what God has done in your life because it was such an amazing feat to overcome. The Israelites, leaving Egypt, saw some of the greatest acts and miracles of God, yet in the wilderness they complained that they had been better off in captivity. They forgot the miracles they experienced because **their focus shifted from the Lord's provision to their circumstances**. You **do not** want to **return to your Egypt!**

Trust in the Lord's goodness to **avoid the trap of ingratitude** and **remorse over loss.** There is always a loss and a gain. **Pursue the more valuable gain.** This life appears valuable but is perishing and worthless. By holding on to this life and old ways, you lose the promised land. To choose the Lord's ways means losing your old way of life. **The life of the believer is a massive exchange program.**

Jesus was everything. He gave up his prominent position to become nothing, carrying the world's burden and becoming our sin. He did this so we could trade in our lives, void of eternal meaning or significance, for an eternal life with position, purpose, and value. **Jesus exchanged His all for our nothing, so we could exchange our nothing for God's all.** What do we gain? We become a vessel containing the spirit of the living, all-powerful God, empowered with all His authority. **You cannot become something until you become nothing.**

Before Paul encountered Jesus, the Pharisees regarded him as a righteous man, yet in God's eyes he was a murderer. After Paul became a follower of Christ, the role switched. He became righteous in God's eyes, but a criminal from the world's point of view. It is best to be seen as nothing by human standards to become everything possible with the Lord.

**Remembrance requires praise.** Praise God for every goodness in your life and all He continues to do. Keep your mind and prayers full of thanksgiving for your transformation, your redemption, and your righteousness. **You cannot be miserable with a heart full of gratitude**, nor can you grumble when **your focus** is on your blessings. Praise is vital to your life as a believer. Praise the Lord through your prayers, your worship, and your testimony. It is the way you enter God's presence. **Praise grabs God's attention**. It keeps your focus off yourself and on Him, keeping you humble and joyful in the Lord, thus giving you strength.

*Enter his gates with thanksgiving, and his courts with praise!*
*Give thanks to him; bless his name! (Psalm 100:4)*

*The Lord is my strength and my shield; in him my heart trusts, and I am helped;*
*my heart exults, and with my song I give thanks to him.*
*(Psalm 28:7)*

*About midnight Paul and Silas were praying and singing hymns to God, and the prisoners were listening to them, and suddenly there was a great earthquake, so that the foundations of the prison were shaken. And immediately all the doors were opened, and everyone's bonds were unfastened.*
*(Acts 16:25 – 26)*

51.11) What have you lost to follow God?

51.12) What have you gained through your relationship with Christ?

51.13) Do you struggle or feel regret or loss for that which you have given up? How?

51.14) Do you believe there is more value in what was gained than what was lost? Why?

51.15) What are you grateful for now? Be specific.

51.16) How do you display your gratitude to God?

## 4. God Moves in Trial

*That I may know him and the power of his resurrection, and may share his sufferings, becoming like him in his death, that by any means possible I may attain the resurrection from the dead. (Philippians 3:10 – 11)*

Jesus experienced every pain common to humanity—persecution, rejection, loss, grief, and fear—yet he never abandoned the Father. Your life should reflect Jesus, in every way, including through times of persecution and trial. It is about the journey and your character, not the outcome. **How you handle a problem is more important than the problem.** Remember God's promises to you and view your struggles from the Lord's perspective. A worldly mindset cannot produce unwavering faith.

It is during life's struggles and trials that we may relapse into old ways, yet it is those same trials that increase our faith and enhance our maturity and closeness with the Lord. **How the trial affects you depends on how you perceive it.** Scripture says to have joy in your trials. Think about how God will work the trial for good.

Joy is eternal, found in God regardless of the circumstance. His Word delights your heart. He is your safe place, your constant standard, never changing, never failing. Joy is the promised end of suffering and the key to standing firm when facing hardship, but how do you have joy when your world is falling apart? In Him, every trial becomes a disguised blessing to rejoice in.

*Though the fig tree should not blossom, nor fruit be on the vines, the produce of the olive fail and the fields yield no food, the flock be cut off from the fold and there be no herd in the stalls, yet I will rejoice in the Lord; I will take joy in the God of my salvation. (Habakkuk 3:17 – 18)*

*Count it all joy, my brothers, when you meet trials of various kinds. (James 1:2)*

*Rejoice in Him! Rejoice in the Lord always; again, I will say, Rejoice. (Philippians 4:4)*

In trials, your joy comes from your hope in the Lord. Unlike false hope in a person, desire, or self, which may fail, **this hope does not depend on a certain outcome**. It trusts God's will and character, believing He is right and has control of the result. God is your refuge, protection, and security. Trust Him. It is when we grow weary of waiting and try to take back control that we stumble.

**Trials end in God's time, not our time**. Do not allow impatience or **seeking a desired outcome** to turn your focus **away from God** and **onto the trial**. Pray constantly, seeking the Lord's truth, guidance, wisdom, and counsel. Search for God's movement in the situation.

*May the God of hope fill you with all joy and peace in believing,*
*so that by the power of the Holy Spirit you may abound in hope. (Romans 15:13)*

*Rejoice in hope, be patient in tribulation, be constant in prayer. (Romans 12:12)*

When our desire is God, He is faithful to give us our desires. If your love and delight are in the Lord, He gives you Himself. **Our desire for a specific result causes worry.** Instead, desire His will to be done. Regardless of how it appears in the moment, you can trust that His outcome is the right answer for every problem. Do not allow troubles in this world to cause you to neglect worship and quiet stillness with the Lord. It is in the secret place, where you sit and enjoy the Lord, that your spirit finds His presence and your joy is full. It is in the Lord that you will find the greatest pleasure, even amid your trials.

*Delight yourself in the Lord, and he will give you the desires of your heart. (Psalm 37:4)*

*You make known to me the path of life; in your presence there is fullness of joy;*
*at your right hand are pleasures forevermore. (Psalm 16:11)*

## Questions to Ponder

51.17) What promises from the Lord should you remember during hard times?

51.18) How can you experience joy in trials?

51.19) How would you describe your desire for the Lord? What do you desire more than Him? This may become a stumbling block in the future.

51.20) How do you have hope when things look impossible?

51.21) Whom in your relationship circles can you lean on when you feel impatient?

51.22) Whom can you depend on to discuss and study Scripture? Who will pray for and with you?

## 5. Move Forward

*Brothers, I do not consider that I have made it my own. But one thing I do: forgetting what lies behind and straining forward to what lies ahead, I press on toward the goal for the prize of the upward call of God in Christ Jesus. (Philippians 3:13 – 14)*

Forgetting what lies behind requires keeping your mind set on forward movement. **Put old ways, old thoughts, and old behaviors to rest** and pursue righteousness. Pressing forward in God's calling on your life cannot include regretting your past or dwelling on what you once had in the world. You cannot forget the person you were, **but as your character transforms, looking more like Christ, the old you will become like a stranger**. Christ defines you; the world no longer has claims on your identity. Your life is no longer your own; a new adventure awaits.

Why do people celebrate a new year? It is a marker in time designated for new beginnings, offering opportunities to start fresh and choose differently. Each new year presents a choice. **You may choose to grieve the loss of the passing year or rejoice in the hope and newness of the unknown and unseen future.** You are embarking on such a season in your life. Will you celebrate the possibilities or grieve the loss of what was?

**The "what if's" in your thoughts can become your downfall**, keeping you stuck in a cycle of emotional turmoil and ineffectiveness. When you try to predict or assume the future, it is like casting a fishing pole to see what bites. What you bait your hook with determines what you will catch. The question "What if I fail?" will set you up for failure. "What if they reject me?" sets you up for rejection. The "what if's" you believe can become self-fulfilling prophecies. This is not the same as New Age positive thinking mantras, by which people believe they have absolute control over what happens to them. But your actions do reflect what you believe, and **what you believe becomes your reality.**

What if you asked different questions? "What if God uses me?" "What if I succeed?" "What if God's Word is true for me?" Your thoughts then become set on success and not failure. You will see alternative possibilities to strive toward, instead of working to avoid scenarios that may not happen. How would your reality change if your self-talk were spoken with confidence as opposed to fear? Fish for victory, not defeat!

<u>Questions to Ponder</u>

51.23) **What old thoughts, behaviors, beliefs, or actions keep resurfacing? Choose to replace them with truth. With what truth will you replace them?**

51.24) **What doubts cause you to ask "what if" questions?**

51.25) **What new questions can you ask yourself when you begin to doubt?**

51.26) **Are there other ways that you may be holding on to your past self?**

6. Keep Growing

*Not that I have already obtained this or am already perfect, but I press on to make it my own, because Christ Jesus has made me his own. ... Let those of us who are mature think this way, and if in anything you think otherwise, God will reveal that also to you. (Philippians 3:12, 15)*

In these verses, Paul acknowledges he is not perfect, but continues to strive for perfection. We too strive for righteousness and perfection, always growing in the Lord. However, **do not think you have "arrived" or understand everything about God**, even as you mature in your faith. Paul also says that if you become prideful in this, God will reveal the truth.

As the Lord speaks to the church of Ephesus,

*But I have this against you, that you have abandoned the love you had at first. Remember therefore from where you have fallen; repent, and do the works you did at first. If not, I will come to you and remove your lampstand from its place, unless you repent.*
*(Revelation 2:2 – 5)*

The church of Ephesus in Revelation seemed to do everything right, but they missed one crucial point. God demanded repentance because they abandoned their love for Him. When our works are no longer done out of Christ's love, but became a religious duty or driven by ambition, they become worthless. **Do not become prideful and forget for whom you work.**

God tells this church to "remember" and "repent." You can think of your journal as a memorial to the mess the Lord has brought you through. The Ephesians church was told to **remember and return to their past works**. They forgot the love and enthusiasm they first had for the Lord when they experienced freedom in Christ. Your journals are not a memorial to your mess, but to the goodness of your God to deliver you. **Continue journaling** your growth in Christ as a record of your freedom. Review your journals often to help remember your love.

It can be easy to fall into the trap of believing you require less study or no longer need to pray before every decision because you now have it all together. You are together because the Lord holds you together and makes you grow. Even as a mentor, you continue learning from the one you disciple. **No matter how much you know, you can always learn from those you lead.**

**Continue to seek the wisdom of your coach.** After *Rebuilt*, you can still benefit from your coach, even if you are coaching others. Allow your coach to continue being the iron that sharpens you, and you will continue to sharpen him or her. God speaks directly to us, yet He designed us to need one another for support, accountability and direction. In His infinite wisdom, God chose to use people to be His ministers and mouthpiece. He will continue to use your coach in your life.

**Once you stop learning and growing, you operate from your own ability.** This is the starting place of pride. God will destroy your pride. The more prideful you are, the more you must endure for Him to reveal your flaws. Stay humble. You will not "arrive" in this life. If Paul, who wrote much of the New Testament, did not arrive, what makes you assume you will (or that you have already done so)? Remember this as your journey continues. The future holds greater understanding for you, as the Lord takes you from one level of glory to the next. Never stop learning. Never stop asking questions and seeking more of God.

## Questions to Ponder

51.27) How will your journaling change after *Rebuilt*?

51.28) Are there a places in your life where you feel you have "arrived"? List them.

51.29) What possible temptations for pride exist in your life now?

51.30) How do you learn from people who are less spiritually mature than you?

51.31) What would you still like to learn about God?

51.32) Where would you like to grow more?

## 7. Cling to the Truth

### *Only let us hold true to what we have attained. (Philippians 3:16)*

The relapse for an alcoholic occurs long before he takes a drink. It begins when his thinking first veers away from what he learned in recovery—possibly weeks before his actions confirm the relapse. The same is true for any issue you are overcoming. Relapse always occurs in the mind first. **The battle to prevent relapse begins with the first thought that is contrary to the truth you have attained.**

If it is difficult for you to catch wrong thinking before it becomes a problem, know it does become easier the longer you walk in truth. No lazy or impulsive mind considers consequences. Stay alert to prevent adverse thoughts from gaining power in your mind.

### The most common gateways to relapse are

- **Pride/control**
- **Temptation**
- **Doubt**
- **Frustration**
- **Fear**
- **Loss/trauma**
- **Fatigue/being overwhelmed**
- **Impulsive behaviors**

When you find yourself faced with any of the above, use the "Stop, Drop, and Roll" exercise from Book One. Immediately take captive any thoughts that contradict, compromise, or conceal the truth and subject those thoughts to God's truth.

Have you ever had a disturbing thought, recognized the lie and dismissed it, just to have the same thought return later? Before you know it, you act as if the thought is true, even though your rational mind knows it is false. Why does this happen? **It is a slow progression from thought to belief.** Positive thinking is not the same as believing truth. The difference involves **a choice.** You must **choose** to believe the truth over the lie. Think of it like flipping on a light switch. When you flip the switch, you are **choosing** to believe God's word and arrest the lie.

There is no other option, God's light switch is either on or off. When false thoughts creep in, **choose** to reject them by turning on the light of God's Word. The goal, of course, is to **always keep the light on**, but it takes a fight of faith to accomplish this.

### Everything is a choice:

✓ **Depressed?** Choose worship.

✓ **Discouraged by others' opinions?** Choose God's truth.

✓ **Anxious?** Choose trust.

✓ **Feeling not good enough?** Choose grace and mercy.

✓ **Angry?** Choose forgiveness.

✓ **Feeling proud or like you need to control a situation?** Choose humility.

✓ **Grumbling or complaining?** Choose praise and gratitude.

✓ **Suffering injustice?** Choose love.

## Questions to Ponder

51.33) Which issues in your life have been the most difficult to overcome?

51.34) How do you respond to each of the gateways to relapse mentioned above?

51.35) How quick are you to notice a detrimental thought?

51.36) What truths will take captive your recurring false thoughts?

51.37) Consider ways you may struggle in the future. How can your coach continue to be a support for you?

# Lesson 52 — Prepare!

## Daily Diligence

The past year has been an intentional movement forward with God, but what happens next week when the daily motivation of this journey ends? Will you return to your old routine?

> *That he [Christ] might sanctify her, having cleansed her by the washing of water with the word, so that he might present the church to himself in splendor, without spot or wrinkle or any such thing, that she might be holy and without blemish. (Ephesians 5:26 – 27)*

> *"Let us rejoice and exult and give him the glory, for the marriage of the Lamb has come, and his Bride has made herself ready; it was granted her to clothe herself with fine linen, bright and pure"—for the fine linen is the righteous deeds of the saints. (Revelation 19:7 – 8)*

You are heading into a season of testing and growth, transforming you into the flawless bride of Christ. Continue with the **same dedication and commitment**. Enter this new season **set apart** for God, seeking to know the Bridegroom more intimately.

## The Mindset of Growth

**Completing *Rebuilt* is not an end but a beginning.** This journey birthed new understanding, introducing God as a Father who raises you up to your ultimate purpose, making you a bride for His Son. Like a toddler, you are learning to walk. You possess the mind of Christ, no longer a mind of flesh or religion. Still, an old stronghold may resurface. You are a spiritual child in a stage of growth. **Reaching maturity in Christ means you grow well, but in this life, you will never stop growing.** How do you grow well? You learn from watching your Father and mimicking Him. You grow because He increases you!

- You do not save yourself. You do not mature yourself, and you cannot fix yourself.
- Your own effort, prayer, study, or work cannot force you to grow in God.
- You grow by knowing the Lord and His character and His ways.
- **You grow through relationship with God.**

Young children grow and learn by watching their parents. As a toddler learning to take steps, you were not thinking about becoming a premier athlete. You did not beat yourself up when you stumbled or fell. You simply stood up and walked again, each step building on the last until your walk became strong. In the end, you learned to run.

Your spiritual walk is like that of the child learning to walk. You cannot learn to walk forward by examining the past or worrying about failures and mistakes. The time for that is over. The purpose of *Rebuilt* was to prepare you to walk forward.

Children spend years watching their parents' behavior and character, and they grow into a portrait of their parents. Like that little child, you must learn by mimicking the actions and character of your Father, observing Him through His Word, His Spirit, and the witness of His people. **As we observe and learn the Lord's character and ways, we transform into the likeness of our heavenly Father.**

## When You Stumble or Fall

Maturity in Christ means **growing well and failing well**. Putting the past behind you does not mean old character flaws will never resurface. God removes our deeply ingrained false beliefs one piece at a time, layer by layer. A person's words or a circumstance may trigger a thought which allows jealousy, fear, control, or insecurity to sneak its way back into your heart. Be careful to avoid the trap of doubt if old behaviors, thoughts, and feelings resurface. Instead of dwelling on your failure, search your heart for the problem the Lord is trying to reveal. Bring it to Him and **continue in a new understanding of an old lesson**.

If the Lord brings a new character issue to light, examine its root, uncover the truth, repent, surrender it, and return to God with a clean slate. **Do not fear more pruning.** Like a stumbling toddler, realize the error, get up, and try again. Never forget you nailed your flaws and failures to the cross. Reject the enemy's lies and move on.

**It is important to recognize trials and failures are a good thing.** Every obstacle teaches a valuable lesson. It is in these moments that our growth is the greatest. Be open to being wrong and reject feelings of insecurity and unworthiness. Instead, ask yourself, **"What is God doing?"** and **"What does this teach me?"**

*For the sake of Christ, then, I am content with weaknesses, insults, hardships, persecutions, and calamities. For when I am weak, then I am strong. (2 Corinthians 12:10)*

Each morning becomes a new opportunity for a **fresh start**. Failure does not mean you have lost the Lord's favor. When you become disillusioned, keep true to who you are in Christ. Stay content, knowing God works everything for your benefit.

*For his anger is but for a moment, and his favor is for a lifetime.*
*Weeping may tarry for the night, but joy comes with the morning. (Psalm 30:5)*

### Questions to Ponder

52.1) Consider the "Mindset of Growth." What are the most important points to apply in your walk with the Lord?

52.2) Are there still strongholds and character flaws with which you struggle?

52.3) Which strongholds or character flaws do you feel you have completely overcome?

52.4) How will you think about future problems, failures, or trials?

## Vision and Plans

*But, as it is written, "What no eye has seen, nor ear heard, nor the heart of man imagined, what God has prepared for those who love him." (1 Corinthians 2:9)*

Where do you see your future? Do you have a desire to serve God's Kingdom stirring in your heart? If you seek His direction and guidance, He will lead each step to fulfill that desire. A life submitted to the Lord's will is greater than your expectations and imaginations, and it will translate into an eternal purpose.

Live out your plans in confidence but **stay flexible for God's detours**. When you are rigid, unwilling to bend past your ideas of what should be, you limit the Lord and your possibilities.

*Commit your work to the Lord, and your plans will be established. (Proverbs 16:2 – 3)*

## Discover Your Calling

God calls every person for one main purpose: to know Him and make Him known. Beyond that, everyone also has a unique purpose for their life and gifts that aid this purpose. People often refer to the latter as their calling. God may call you into a specific occupation, role, or ministry, but it is your relationship with Him that paves the way to a more fulfilling life. So how do you find your specific calling? **The simple answer is you don't.** Your calling finds you.

When God calls you into a ministry, He makes it quite clear. He prepares the way forward and readies your heart and character for the challenges ahead. If you try to jump into your calling unprepared, you may fall into pride. People who serve in ministry roles often fail because they get caught up in pride, mistaking their anointing for their own skill and ability. Their pride may lead to other sins, such as sexual or financial sins. **Be careful not to get stuck on a title, ministry, how your role appears, or how quickly it should grow.** Do not overthink it. Walk with the Lord. He will guide you, one step at a time, toward success.

*<u>Do not despise these small beginnings</u>, for the LORD rejoices to see the work begin, to see the plumb line in Zerubbabel's hand. (Zechariah 4:10, NLT)*

Allow your life to become a living testimony of God. The Lord sets you apart as His ambassador, to represent Him. The world watches you closely with curiosity and skepticism. The words and actions of every believer display a picture of God to them. **If you look like everyone else but claim the gospel message, they see a hypocrite. If you look like Jesus, they see the truth of God in you.**

God often calls people into a ministry that makes use of their talents and gifting. Are you an artist? Your art can glorify God. Jesus does not call everyone to serve in church ministry, but He calls every believer to be a witness and light to a dark world. Your witness is no less valuable in your workplace, home, hobbies, or civic service. Are you a songwriter, a carpenter, a graphic designer, a mechanic? Each of these skills can benefit God's Kingdom and may become your ministry, but **sometimes your calling is completely unrelated to your abilities**.

God's calling on your life may relate to an area where the enemy attacks you most. Satan loves to preempt a move of God. A socially awkward person may become a pastor. A person insecure in their words may become a mouthpiece for God. The teen kicked out of school, unable to graduate, may become a professional author. The bossy know-it-all, ridiculed their entire life, may become a prominent leader. The selfish business executive may give his life to help people in need. **It is in our weaknesses that we find our greatest strengths in God.**

Moses was not seeking to be the deliverer of Israel when God sent him; he was simply curious about a bush that was on fire but did not burn. Moses was not trying to become the Moses we read about in Scripture. He just obeyed God, and God used his life to prepare him for what he was to become. **You do not need all the answers.** The important thing is to keep growing in the Lord.

It may be awkward at first to walk in your true calling, but soon the calling will feel like home. As God calls you into your purpose and equips you for success, you will discover there is nothing in the world you would rather do. **Stay open-minded to his plans.**

It can be tempting to **create a calling** for yourself **or usurp another person's calling** as your own. The book of Numbers tells the story of Korah, a Levite during the time of Moses and Aaron. God appointed the Levites for all the tabernacle service, but this honor did not satisfy Korah. He was envious of Aaron, chosen as the high priest. Korah's jealousy and envy of a calling that did not belong to him brought a rebellion that ended his ministry and his life.

How can you receive a calling that God has set aside for another? If you are seeking to be an evangelist but God called you to be a youth minister, you may function as an evangelist but fail to prosper in that role. When you stop pursuing a blessing that belongs to another and pursue your true purpose, you will receive the Lord's full blessings. **You cannot become who God created you to be if you are acting like someone you are not.**

## Appoint Your Days

*So teach us to number our days, that we may get a heart of wisdom. (Psalm 90:12)*

This verse speaks about using our time productively because our days on earth are few. But this does **not** imply that you should become busier. Rather, it speaks to how you spend time. The word for numbering in Hebrew is *manah*. It means to appoint, reckon, or count. Numbering your days speaks to appointing or **purposing** each day for the Lord. Your life set apart for the Lord means **your time belongs to Him**. The reward is a heart of wisdom.

Each day offers new opportunity and purpose. **How you start off your morning sets the tone for your day.** It can transform your perspective and prepare your heart for whatever comes. Before your feet hit the floor, give the Lord your attention, your day, your prayers, and worship. **Consecrate each day to the Lord, dedicating it for His purposes.**

Numbering your days is more than making plans; it is making every moment of every day purposely dedicated to Him. **Each moment presents a choice** to do or not do something. **Every choice follows one of two paths**: to walk God's path or follow the ways of the world. Let the Lord direct your every thought, word, and step. He opens doors and exposes wrong choices.

*But seek first the kingdom of God and his righteousness, and all these things will be added to you. (Matthew 6:33)*

Be careful how you choose to spend your time and consider for whom you are spending it. The world distracts you with **worthless pursuits** that steal your time and attention. Anything that indulges this world and its values is worthless. Limit worthless pursuits. A **worthwhile pursuit** progresses your relationship with God and your calling or purpose. Ask yourself, "Does this benefit the purpose God gave me?"

*You adulterous people! Do you not know that friendship with the world is enmity with God? Therefore whoever wishes to be <u>a friend of the world makes himself an enemy of God</u>. (James 4:4)*

*Therefore, my beloved brothers, <u>be steadfast, immovable, always abounding in the work of the Lord</u>, knowing that in the Lord your labor is not in vain. (1 Corinthians 15:58)*

*Whoever works his land will have plenty of bread, but*
*he who follows worthless pursuits lacks sense. (Proverbs 12:11)*

Which activities in your normal day are worthwhile pursuits? Fun activities with your children or spouse may appear frivolous but may also enhance those relationships. However, if you are seeking fun to gratify the flesh with entertainment, your priorities could be wrong. Pray and use discernment to determine if your pursuits are in line with God's will.

*Whatever you do, work at it with your whole being, for the Lord and not for men.*
*(Colossians 3:23, BSB)*

---

<u>Questions to Ponder</u>

52.5)   What does it mean to prepare your days to walk with the Lord?

52.6)   How will setting apart your day change the choices you make throughout the day?

52.7)   Considering the vision, calling, and purpose the Lord has shown you for your life, what tasks would you consider *worthwhile* pursuits?

52.8)   Examine your normal activities for the day. Which are *worthless* pursuits?

*52.9)*   What activities are *ignoble*, neither worthwhile nor worthless? (This includes necessary, mundane tasks.)

52.10) Examine your motives for Christian activities (i.e., prayer, worship, serving, and studying). Are you seeking to earn the Lord's approval, or to know Him more?

---

## Negotiables and Non-negotiables

It is never easy to appoint your days for God while balancing life's obligations. Are you a person who schedules every minute of your day? Or is routine difficult for you? Does an incomplete to-do list discourage you? If allowing the Lord to guide your day seems impossible under the burden and demands of life, **it is time to reexamine your tasks**.

**Make two lists**

Flexibility allows time for God's unexpected plans and divine appointments, yet there are some tasks you should never neglect. List your **non-negotiable** tasks, things you must do regardless of what happens. This is a very brief list that only includes "worthwhile pursuits." For a believer, this list **will include** personal time with God, prayer, worship, studying Scripture, and journaling. You may have other commitments that you consider non-negotiable, such as specific special moments with your family, praying with your children before bed, or even a family game night.   Your non-negotiable list **does not include** meetings, routines, or appointments on your calendar. You may reschedule these if something or someone else needs your time. Therefore, although they may be a high priority, they *are* negotiable and not mandatory.

Everything **not** on this list is **negotiable**, including meetings, phone calls, social media, videos or television, appointments, your worthless pursuits, and sometimes even baths and sleep. **Negotiable tasks are flexible.** Think differently about what you must do. Some negotiables may seem mandatory, such as meal preparation. Of course, you must eat, but **when** you eat may be flexible, or you can plan a simple dinner in a pinch. List your negotiable daily tasks and activities.

Finally, **prioritize the negotiable list**. Think of this list as your daily "to-do" list. Sort this list by items most important to complete. Your non-negotiable and negotiable lists will rarely change, but you may need to review your priorities daily. A low priority one day may become a foremost priority the next day as your situation changes.

**Use your lists**
The goal of a non-negotiable list is to make you **less busy**. The important, life-altering tasks will take priority over every other task. After finishing the non-negotiables, complete any tasks on your negotiable list in your remaining time. **Negotiables never replace non-negotiables** and are always subject to the Lord's plans for your day. To live this way **lightens your schedule for unexpected situations** that require your attention.

**It is important not to skimp on non-negotiables to allow for negotiable tasks.** Your non-negotiables will become routine or obligatory if your schedule restricts their available time so you can fit in all your negotiable tasks. Remember, the Lord's timing is perfect. You truly do not need to accomplish everything you think you do.

If, for example, you limit your quiet time with the Lord to a specific time frame, your focus will divert to the time and obligation of your prayer, rather than the prayer itself. How much revelation can you receive when you cut short your time studying the Word? Is it possible to determine how much time you should worship God, how long you speak to Him, or the time He has available to speak to you? Try not to restrict God's time. When seeking the Lord becomes routine, like making an appointment with the Lord, **it is like checking off a religious duty instead of enjoying a relationship**.

## I Can't Do That!
You may believe you are too busy to give God unlimited time, but this is not true. Martin Luther once said, "If I fail to spend two hours in prayer each morning, the devil gets the victory through the day." The enemy would distract, interrupt, and distort him from his purpose. He also said, "I have so much to do that I shall spend the first three hours in prayer." The Lord focused his mind and established his plans for the day. Martin Luther knew he needed to give the Lord time first to accomplish all he needed. He is not alone. Many prominent (and busy) people claim they pray for hours each morning to be productive.

Sometimes your mind will fight against the non-negotiables. Even when you struggle, you can pray, worship, or read Scripture. Often when we do not "feel like it," we actually need it most. Be obedient. **Half the battle is beginning**, and the "feeling like it" will come.

> ### Questions to Ponder
> **52.11) Create a list of the non-negotiables in your life. Keep this list minimal. Many things that are important to you are still negotiable.**

**52.12)** Create a list of negotiable activities in your normal day. This should be a generic list. (Instead of listing every appointment, you could simply list the type of appointment, such as work meetings, doctor appointments, *Rebuilt* meetings, church functions, etc.)

**52.13)** From your negotiable list, choose 3 items that are the highest priority. (When choosing, think, "If I cannot do anything else today, I will do this.")

**52.14)** Bring your lists to the Lord. Seek His heart about them. Do you feel there is something God wants you to add or remove from the non-negotiable list? Is there anything He wants you to make a higher priority?

## Obligation and Distraction

One of the hardest things to surrender may be your schedule, especially if you have a family and children. **We often treat unnecessary things like requirements.** God knows the tasks we should and should not do. Give Him your days because His timing is perfect, and His plan is flawless.

**God is not in a hurry; why are you?** His plan will keep you busy, but His leading does not make you feel driven. The Lord may put an urgency in your heart, but if you seem rushed or pressured, it is likely your flesh, other people, or the enemy, not God.

People often put their needs or expectations on your days. Intentionally or not, people take advantage and disrespect your time. **The ability to say "No" is the most important lesson you can learn.** You should not do something simply because you can. People's expectations must take second place to your non-negotiables and to the Lord. Plenty of time is available for needed tasks, but not always for expected tasks. **Your responsibility is to God's checklist**, not to the desires of family, friends, and neighbors. Your non-negotiables must take precedence over everything else, keeping you flexible to minister where the Lord sends you. **Listen for the Lord to direct you to whom you should help and how.**

To allow pressure, demands, phone calls, social media, distractions, or other confusion to rob you of those most important things **will** cause you to lose focus. Take your negotiable tasks to the Lord and let His timing prevail. A delay rarely becomes a serious problem, although people may make it seem that way.

1. **Slow down.** God is not in a hurry. His plans never fail.

2. **Do not limit God's time.** Nothing is more important than your relationship with Him.

3. **Trust God.** It is okay if something does not get done. God knows your responsibilities, commitments, and desires. All things happen in God's perfect timing.

4. **Let God lead.** We can easily get distracted from the tasks we should do.

52.15)  What things or activities distract you from what you should do?

52.16)  Which people in your life distract you from what you should do?

52.17)  To whom do you have difficulty saying "No"?

52.18)  Do you feel pressured, hurried, or driven? What or who causes these feelings?

52.19)  How will you slow down?

## Test Everything

*Test everything; hold fast what is good. Abstain from every form of evil.*
*(1 Thessalonians 5:21 – 22)*

Testing everything is more than testing spirits; it is testing your words and deeds and the words and deeds of others. Were the messages you heard today founded on truth? Stay true to what the Lord has shown you. Do not waver and do not doubt.

Check your heart throughout the day and in the evening. Where did you doubt? What temptations did you have? How did you handle mistakes? How did you do **well**? What frivolous activities did you engage in? Did you make progress? Can you do better?

*But if we judged ourselves truly, we would not be judged. But when we are judged by the Lord, we are disciplined so that we may not be condemned along with the world.*
*(1 Corinthians 11:31)*

**Judge yourself honestly and you will not be judged.** We are tested in our weakness. Guard your mind at all costs and keep your eyes focused on the Lord. Be honest with yourself about the true condition of your heart. **Denial is Satan's best friend.** It is when we are too afraid or ashamed to admit our faults that the enemy sets us up for disaster. When we are honest about our weakness, the Lord works in it and transforms it into our greatest strength.

When you examine the truth of your heart and honestly see your sin, you can give it to the Lord. Avoiding issues keeps you buried under hidden shame. Admitting mistakes allows you to correct them, seek forgiveness, and keep going. It is good to experience the gravity of your wrongs. Without remorse, you will continue in or return to the sin. **Likewise, it is good to learn from your errors, forgive yourself, and put it behind you.** God renews us after we fall. **Why would you continue punishing yourself?**

## Questions to Ponder

52.20)  How well do you recognize your failings and sin?

52.21)  Tell how the Lord has used past failures for your benefit.

52.22)  Do you feel you must punish yourself or continue dwelling on past wrongs? Why?

*(Continue to the Daily Heart Check.)*

## Daily Heart Check

A good way to judge yourself honestly is with a daily heart check. Contemplate your day each evening as you journal. Search your heart for wrongs you have done and ways you have walked righteously. Keep your eyes on the Lord regardless of what is happening around you. Continue having the mind of Christ, your love and thoughts unified with the Lord.

*Purge me with hyssop, and I shall be clean; wash me, and I shall be whiter than snow. Let me hear joy and gladness; let the bones that you have broken rejoice. Hide your face from my sins and blot out all my iniquities. Create in me a clean heart, O God, and renew a right spirit within me. (Psalm 51:8)*

*So if there is any encouragement in Christ, any comfort from love, any participation in the Spirit, any affection and sympathy, complete my joy by being of the same mind, having the same love, being in full accord and of one mind. (Philippians 2:1 – 2)*

1. **In the morning** – Begin your day by consecrating it for the Lord's purposes. Pray, worship, and study.

2. **Throughout the day** – Seek the Lord every moment and choose His ways in each decision. Guard your mind to keep the mind of Christ.

3. **In the evening** – Journal about your day and perform a short heart check. Thank the Lord for your blessings and the work he is doing in your heart through your trials.

**The following questions may help you evaluate your day and check your heart.**

- Was there conflict today? Did I ignore it or address it? What in my heart may have led me to see this issue incorrectly?

- In what situations did I fail today? In what ways did I place confidence in my ability apart from the Lord?

- How did I do well today? Where did I have confidence in God's work through me?

- Am I thankful for something I used to take for granted?

- How was I distracted? Are distractions taking from more important things? How can I solve this issue?

- Has something occurred today that brought forth regret, discontent, or ingratitude?

- Am I worried? Where is the hope in this situation?

- Did I have patience and seek the Lord as I walked through my day?

- How did I grow in the Lord today?

- Did I have pride today, or did I try to control a circumstance? Did I doubt God?

- Was I tempted today?

- Did I feel (and how did I handle) fear, insecurity, frustration, fatigue, or being overwhelmed?

- Is a major issue happening in my life right now? Am I trusting God for the outcome? Am I seeking the Lord for wisdom and giving Him control?

- What is God showing and teaching through my trials today? Am I trusting Him in the trials?

## Your Final Assignment

The most important part of your recovery is writing and sharing your testimony. Your testimony is the reality of God's goodness, shown through your personal story. Sharing truth learned, and the experience of being set free by that truth, draws others to Christ.

In the Scripture stories, when people experienced God's miraculous work, they built an altar to the Lord. Noah came off the ark and built an altar. God gave land to Abraham, and he built an altar. God gave Isaac land with a promise to multiply his descendants, and Isaac built an altar. **Scripture contains many such examples of altars and memorials to the Lord.**

God knows people's memories are short. Memorials help His people remember His goodness and love for them. The enemy also knows man's fickleness. He knows the farther you are from your victories, the easier it is to forget the wilderness you came from and the miracles throughout the journey.

Memorials in Scripture come in many forms: feasts, altars, writings, and Scripture itself. Communion is also a memorial, a way to remember the sacrifice Jesus made for us. Your journals serve as a memorial of your wilderness journey with the Lord. **Your testimony is another memorial—your gift back to the Lord.**

Which brings us to your last assignment. You will build a memorial, a story of remembrance for everything the Lord has done in your life. This will not be an altar of brick and stone, but one forged from the sweat and tears of your journey.

*And he took bread, and when he had given thanks, he broke it and gave it to them, saying, "This is my body, which is given for you. <u>Do this in remembrance of me</u>."*
*(Luke 22:19)*

*Truly, I say to you, wherever this gospel is proclaimed in the whole world, what she has done will also be told <u>in memory of her</u>. (Matthew 26:13)*

*Then the Lord said to Moses, "<u>Write this as a memorial in a book</u> and recite it in the ears of Joshua, that I will utterly blot out the memory of Amalek from under heaven." <u>And Moses built an altar and called the name of it, The Lord Is My Banner.</u>*
*(Exodus 17:14 – 15)*

*That this be a sign among you, so that when your children ask later, saying, "What do these stones mean to you?", then you shall say to them, "Because the waters of the Jordan were cut off before the ark of the covenant of the Lord; when it crossed the Jordan, the waters of the Jordan were cut off." So <u>these stones shall become a memorial to the sons of Israel forever</u>. (Joshua 4:4 – 7)*

*So these days were to be remembered and celebrated throughout every generation, every family, every province and every city; and these days of Purim were not to fail from among the Jews, <u>or their memory fade</u> from their descendants. (Esther 9:28)*

*Now this <u>day will be a memorial to you</u>, and you shall celebrate it as a feast to the Lord; throughout your generations you are to celebrate it as a permanent ordinance.*
*(Exodus 12:14)*

## Turn Your History into His Story

Rewrite your life story from the truth that the Lord has revealed to you. Your story will become a place to draw strength and truth. When you slip into old thinking, your story will serve to remind you of the Lord's transformative work. For others, it will become a testimony of encouragement, and a witness to the unbeliever. Use the guidelines that follow to rewrite your story and then share it with your coach.

- Gather your journals from your *Rebuilt* journey. Reread them. What you read will amaze you; it is worth the effort!

- Use your lists from your inventory to create a timeline of major events in your life.

- Write out the story of what happened during each life event.

- For each life event, write the truth as you now understand it.

  o Where was God in the event?

  o How did God use this event to benefit you or others?

- Mention how you felt then and describe your feelings now that you understand the truth!

## Go!

Jesus gave us a great commission to make disciples. We are all expected by God to minister in the lives of others. He equips us with gifts and talents to help His Kingdom grow, but *Rebuilders* have something many do not have: a powerful testimony! Your coach can help you shorten your story to make a great testimony or pull from parts of your story to minister to someone's specific need. Even if your calling is not with *Rebuilt*, your testimony will be a powerful witness wherever the Lord leads you.

### Serving with *Rebuilt*

If everyone who completes *Rebuilt* will coach only one person, the impact would be exponential. Your journey has equipped you to serve others and witness their lives transform as well. You continue growing even more when walking with another on their journey.

- We ask everyone who has completed their *Rebuilt* journey to write and share a video testimony to encourage others on their journey. You may choose how and where you share your testimony.

- Consider becoming a *Rebuilt* coach. We have training and materials available if you would like to lead others on a journey. The amazing thing about leading others is that you continue to grow right along with them!

- Consider becoming an online coach, guiding those who take the journey online.

- Consider joining the leadership team with *Rebuilt*. (You must first become a coach.)

<u>Questions to Ponder</u>

52.23) Rewrite your story and share it with your coach.

52.24) Do you have questions or concerns about sharing your testimony?

52.25) Do you see yourself serving with *Rebuilt*? How?

52.26) Write any questions you have for your coach about continuing forward.

Ask your coach for information about opportunities to serve with *Rebuilt!*

# Appendix

## Contents

# How to Have Confidence

How can you be confident moving forward? The answer is not dependent on who you are, specific to a denomination, based on your gifts, your talents, or your success rate. Your confidence is based on and in the Lord, who has all knowledge and power. He gives gifts and talent to everyone,

You can find confidence in the power and purpose behind your abilities. The power comes from the Lord, and the purpose is His will. Those whose confidence lies in their talents or gifts are missing the One who enables the gifting. This is a counterfeit confidence.

The question is never "Are you able?" Rather it is "Do you have confidence in the God who makes you able?" When you have the master instructing you, is there anything you cannot do?

Picture a woman who fumbles around the kitchen, barely able to fix a simple meal. Her daughter is having a large graduation party and wants her to cook an enormous dinner for everyone. Yet the woman has never cooked such an elaborate meal.

Terrified, she realizes she does not have the money to hire a caterer for the party. But she knows a master chef, and she calls him for advice. He tells her everything she needs to buy, how to prepare the food, which seasonings to add, and how to cook it.

Now the woman has every confidence in her ability to fix the dinner. However, her confidence is not in her own talent but in the ability of the master chef guiding her.

**To lack confidence in yourself is to lack confidence in God, the one guiding you through life.** He is the master of everything, and there is nothing He cannot lead you through!

# Battling Pride

*I love photography! It is my favorite hobby, and one I wanted to make a career. Before shooting an event, I met with the client and asked questions until I had a detailed understanding of the final product they desired.*

*I knew precisely what they wanted before setting the stage for the shoot. Then, I began preparing the setting, creating the mood, and choosing the poses that would make my clients' photos into treasured and irreplaceable memories. My talent was often praised as I found beauty in the ordinary and captured those spontaneous moments that would otherwise be forever lost.*

*Why did I abandon my aspiration to be a professional photographer? Because it is exhausting! My clients constantly argued with me, pompously touting their flawed theories of how the stage should be set, what would work, and what I should do. They grumbled and complained, thinking they knew better how to produce the desired results.*

*But I was the photographer. I had the knowledge and experience. I knew the lighting, angles, and poses. I knew what they should wear and how they should stand. I understood the subtleties that make a photo great. After all, that was the reason they hired me.*

*This fictional scenario illustrates a truth in our relationship with God. He knows the beginning and the end and all that falls between. He knows how everything works because He created it all. Is there anything He can't do? Yet we argue and complain, thinking that His way will not provide the desired results. We think we know better than the professional and want it done our way. The Lord set the stage and put every piece in place. It is our job to swallow our pride and get out of His way.*

# Choose Your Diet

The problem with most diets is the nature of the diet. A diet designed for rapid transformation causes radical changes to the way you eat and live. But these changes are not sustainable. You cannot physically or mentally continue eating the same way. Eventually you will lose progress, regressing into old habits.

The perfect diet is one that alters your lifestyle. It doesn't leave you hungry or deprived. It is based on sustainability and balance. A good diet alters the way you eat forever. The changes are not as rapid, but you will find them permanent.

**Jesus said to them, "I am the bread of life; whoever comes to me shall not hunger, and whoever believes in me shall never thirst. (John 6:35)**

**Consider your transformation with God like the perfect diet.** You are eating the bread of life and drinking water that never leaves you thirsty. You experience breakthroughs that must be tested and tried so they become a solid, sustainable, change in you. Balance takes time. Remember, the urge you feel to rush back to the world's junk food is a test to strengthen you and bring your transformation to completion.

**More than that, we rejoice in our sufferings, knowing that suffering produces endurance, and endurance produces character, and character produces hope. (Romans 5:3-4)**

Don't try to run ahead of God! Expecting your first victory to be the end all, is like eating a fad diet. Seeking instant gratification leads to a superficial walk with Jesus. When it seems like you are being tested again and again, do not fall into frustration, condemnation, or shame. Have joy! God is molding you into His likeness. Embrace the process. Stop fighting Him! You can't change yourself, but God can. And your acceptance and cooperation make the process much easier.

The authentic work of God is not instant gratification,
rather it is sustainable and eternal.

Want the Real Thing!

# Passing the Test

Scripture says that we are tested through our trials and tribulations. What does this mean? Why would God test us, and how do we know if we pass or fail a test? We find the answer in the book of Job.

*And if they are bound in chains and caught in the cords of affliction, then he declares to them their work and their transgressions, that they are behaving arrogantly. He opens their ears to instruction and commands that they return from iniquity... He delivers the afflicted by their affliction and opens their ear by adversity. He also allured you out of distress into a broad place where there was no cramping, and what was set on your table was full of fatness. (Job 8 – 10, 15 – 16)*

In this passage, Elihu explains how the Lord uses our trials. Job experienced some of the hardest trials depicted in Scripture. He did not understand why, as a righteous man, he was suffering so much pain and loss. His wife told him to curse God and die, and his friends tried to convince him that his suffering was due to some sin, so he should simply repent. Instead of defending the Lord's righteousness in the situation, Job began to defend his righteousness to the people accusing him of wrongdoing. Despite his grief and pain, he was concerned with the opinions of man, and thus he became lifted in pride. Then Elihu comes forth and speaks truth to Job, leading him to repentance and restoration.

From Elihu's message to Job, we can see that God uses the trials, temptations, and tribulations we face to get our attention. When we are prepared to listen, He shows us the iniquity in our hearts. The Lord speaks through the chains of our affliction and opens our ears to hear his words through adversity. Then, when we have learned from the test, the Lord can restore and bless us.

That which seems like failure, is a growing process. The only way to fail is if the test does not result in understanding and growth. We will continue to be tested through adversity until we are perfected in our character.

*For you know that the testing of your faith produces steadfastness. And let steadfastness have its full effect, that you may be perfect and complete, lacking in nothing. (James 1:3 – 4)*

# Fear vs Truth

*He who has an ear, let him hear! Do you ever feel defeated, condemned? Do you ever ask yourself, "What is wrong with me?", "Why am I going through this again?", or "Why do I keep failing?". Do you still feel like God's word is truth for other people, but not for you? Or, perhaps, you feel like God is not the problem, but you are. You just are too messed up or too bad for God to fix.*

*If you have any of these thoughts, you likely have shame. Remember, guilt is when you have done something bad, but shame is when you believe you are bad. We all have a sin nature that makes us wicked. The truth is that Jesus died to overcome our sin. We do not own that identity.*

*God calls you righteous through your faith, your repentance, and the blood of Jesus. He has given you a purpose, a future, and a hope.* **But how can He use someone for His kingdom, who feels like they are unqualified to be used?**

| **FEAR** | **TRUTH** |
|---|---|
| **F** – *False* | **T** – *True* |
| **E** – *Evidence* | **R** – *Reality* |
| **A** – *Appearing* | **U** – *Unfolding* |
| **R** – *Real* | **T** – *Through* |
| | **H** - *Him* |

*You must come out of agreement with the lies. You can choose to believe what God says is good and evil or choose to believe your own ideas of good and evil.* **Who are you to say you are bad when God says you are righteous?**

**It is the Holy Spirit's job to convict you of sin.** *The enemy's tactic is to cause you to doubt and question "What if I can't see what's wrong with me or if I am wrong?"* **Don't seek the wrong, seek the Lord.** *He will bring your sin to your attention. Once he shows you, it is your job to repent from it and allow Him to correct it. God is faithful to finish what He started in you! Ask God if there is any way in you that displeases Him and trust Him to reveal it to you. It is not your job to discover what the Spirit has not revealed.*

# The Choice of Two

**<u>See, I have set before you today life and goodness, as well as death and disaster.</u>**
*For I am commanding you today to love the LORD your God, to walk in His ways, and to keep His commandments, statutes, and ordinances, so that you may live and increase, and the LORD your God may bless you in the land that you are entering to possess. But if your heart turns away and you do not listen, but are drawn away to bow down to other gods and worship them, I declare to you today that you will surely perish; you shall not prolong your days in the land that you are crossing the Jordan to possess. I call heaven and earth as witnesses against you today that* **<u>I have set before you life and death, blessing and cursing. Therefore choose life,</u>** *so that you and your descendants may live. (Deuteronomy 30:15-19 BSB)*

*God does not change.*

*For I the Lord do not change… (Malachi 3:6)*

*Jesus Christ is the same yesterday and today and forever. (Hebrews 13:8)*

*The counsel of the Lord stands forever, the plans of his heart to all generations. (Psalm 33:11)*

Choose life and live or choose death and cursing. This is the same choice presented to the first man and woman. The choice represented by two trees in the center of the garden. Choose the first, the Tree of Life, from which eternal life flowed, or choose the Tree of the Knowledge of Good and Evil, which led to death and separation from God. This is the choice He presented the Israelites as they entered the promised land. **God offers us the same choice today,** that He has given humanity since the beginning of our existence.

In the garden, mankind had dominion over everything, yet **there was one thing that God never allowed mankind to do – to decide for themselves what was good and evil.** He was the author of good, and He alone defined it.

The way the story is told in children's storybooks may make you think that this tree had some magical power to instantly reveal knowledge of good and evil by eating its fruit, but that is not exactly what happened.

**<u>When the woman saw that the tree was good</u>** **for food and <u>pleasing to the eyes</u>, and that <u>it was desirable</u> for obtaining wisdom, she took the fruit and ate it. She also gave some to her husband who was with her, and he ate it. (Genesis 3:6-7)**

At that moment, doubting God's truth, the woman decided she knew the tree was good. She decided that what she thought was good and desirable was better than what God thought was good and desirable, and it led to a curse and the death of her sinless nature. Her choice was pride, lack of faith, lack of trust, leaning on her own understanding, and blatant sin – disobedience to God. These are the same things we struggle with today.

*Each moment of each day we are presented with the choice to choose life and live.*

Everything we deal with in this life can be boiled down to the same choice. Do we choose our own idols and desires, that which we want and think is good, or do we choose what God says is good and trust His thoughts and understanding regarding what is right?

Galatians 5 shows us the contrast between acts that come from God's way of thinking and our sin nature's way of thinking. If we think in our flesh (sin nature) we choose death. If we choose the mind of Christ, we choose life!

**The acts of the flesh are obvious: sexual immorality, impurity, and debauchery; idolatry and sorcery; hatred, discord, jealousy, and rage; rivalries, divisions, factions, and envy; drunkenness, orgies, and the like. I warn you, as I did before, that those who practice such things will not inherit the kingdom of God. But the fruit of the Spirit is love, joy, peace, patience, kindness, goodness, faithfulness, gentleness, and self-control. Against such things there is no law. (Galatians 5:19-22)**

Sorcery is attempting to make what you want to happen in your power (or Satan's power). Hatred is something you don't want or like. Discord is creating problems to get your way. Jealousy is the fear of losing what is yours to another. Rage and anger burn in your heart when you become offended. **All of these things allow your own desires and understanding to define what is good, instead of believing what God says is good**.

We are not much different than the serpent, quick to twist God's truth to fit our circumstances and desires. Therefore we must take off the ways of our old life and old ways of thinking and put on the mind of Christ. We must not lean on our understanding, but acknowledge God in all our ways, and take every thought and feeling captive and make it obedient to Christ.

**God alone had the right to determine good and evil.** He alone is just, and His justice is right. When we do not agree with His actions – **HE IS RIGHT.** When we decide for ourselves how things should or should not be, or what is or is not good **we are trying to take the place of God and usurp His authority.**

When we value something as more important (better) than God or His ways we choose death. When we set aside our own desires and wisdom to follow God, His commandments, and His ways, we choose life. Not sure which choice you are making? Examine your fruit! What do you do when you don't get what you want, or when things don't go how you think they should go? What do you do when you are frustrated because things are hard and you are impatient?

*Choose to believe God is good and trust in the goodness of His ways.*
*It's just that simple!*

# The Root of All Emotion

We have an enemy that loves to play on the emotions of our sin nature, and a God who is trying to transform our sin nature into one that looks like Him. We are caught in a war of thoughts, a battle between God and Satan fighting for our soul.

Think of it as if you are the object of a huge custody battle with two parents each demanding full right to you, each claiming you belong to them. Every day, the devil stands before the court making accusations, testifying of all the ways you mess up and all the reasons you belong to him. He has gone to great lengths to tempt you to reject God and His ways. **Satan is fear** and **lies.**

On the other side of the court, Jesus stands with the custody documents. He owns you and your debt has been paid in full. The cost, His life. He counters every argument of the enemy with your righteousness, all your wrongs justified for a price. **God is love**, a parent who is just and deals only in **truth.**

Our emotions send us messages that catch us up in a war of thoughts between these two opposites. Messages that bounce between truth and lies, depending on their source, distorting God's truth with a twisted understanding that leaves us double minded. It is hard to see truth clearly when our emotions seem to confirm the enemy's convincing lies.

Of course, it's complicated... Or is it?

In psychology, there is a claim that **every emotion we feel, is rooted in one of two sources, either love or fear**. This aligns with scripture. Emotions speak messages to your mind. An emotion rooted in love comes from the Lord and is truth, and an emotion rooted in fear comes from the enemy and is a lie. It may seem simple to identify from which source an emotion flows, but **many times it is not.** Therefore, we must take emotions captive, examine them, and submit them to the word of God, and never rely on them to guide our thoughts and actions.

Anger is an emotion that you may quickly identify as being rooted in fear, but God says in scripture to love what he loves and hate what he hates, and God himself gets angry. Scripture says not to be angry because the anger of man is not righteous, and also to be angry — but not sin in your anger. This is because Anger **can come from either source.**

*How do you win the battle of your emotions? Be perfected in Love!*

**So we have come to know and to believe the love that God has for us. God is love, and whoever abides in love abides in God, and God abides in him. By this is love perfected with us, so that we may have confidence for the day of judgment, because as he is so also are we in this world. There is no fear in love, but perfect love casts out fear. For fear has to do with punishment, and whoever fears has not been perfected in love. We love because he first loved us. (1 John 4:16-19)**

### Three ways to find the source of your emotion

1. **To find the source ask yourself why?**
   If the reason for your emotion lines up with God's thoughts and ways, it is likely based in love.  If not, it may be based in fear.
   Here are a couple of examples.

   - **Why am I angry?**
     Are you angry at unrighteousness, or was there a true injustice?  Were God or His ways being disrespected? This anger may be rooted in love.
     Did something not go your way? Did you dislike an outcome or result?  Did someone make you feel bad or insecure?  This is anger probably based in fear.

   - **Why do I love?**
     Is my love for a person sacrificial? Is it patient and slow to anger, kind and not self-seeking? Do I love because I want to grow with another in God, give myself, invest my time, and share my life and resources with them? This love is based out of God's love.
     Do I love them because they have a lot in common with me and they fill a missing spot in my life? Because I don't want to be lonely, or they fill a lack in my life? Am I looking for something specific from them like protection or security? Do they fill a need? This love may be based out of fear.

   - **Why do I feel proud?**
     Is my confidence because I know God makes me able, or in the quality of person God is transforming in me? If your confidence is in the Lord, it is based in Love.
     God warns against pride. Do you feel a need to boast or put others down to make yourself appear better? Do you feel insecure? Do you fear failing? Do you think you are entitled? Do you need to prove yourself? Are you trying to be good enough?  Do you think others are not as good as you? This is fear-based pride.

2. **To find the source examine the message you hear in your mind.**
   Do the messages you hear make you feel loved, love others, feel compassion, have joy, give you confidence or purpose? These are messages from love.
   Do the messages make you feel defeated, hopeless, fearful, or condemned? Are they selfish thoughts or do they appeal to your flesh? Do you feel like a failure, or fear the opinions of man? These are messages based in fear.

3. **To find the source examine your fruit, the actions, that result from your thoughts and emotions.**
   Do your actions bring glory to the Lord? Do they build others up and biblically cover their sin? Do they follow God's commandments? They are love-based.
   Do they cause others harm or tear people down? Do they puff you up with pride? Do they indulge your flesh? These are based in fear.

# I Shall Not Want

Why did God's people in the Old Testament continually turn to false gods, even though the Lord was faithful to them? He gave them astounding victories over their enemies, blessings, and riches. In the wilderness, their clothes did not wear out and provision fell from the sky. Yet, they were never satisfied, always wanting, serving other gods and idols trying to satisfy the desires of their flesh. This angered God.

> **Because you did not serve the LORD your God <u>with joyfulness and gladness of heart</u>, because of the abundance of all things, you shall serve your enemies in hunger and thirst, in nakedness, and lacking everything. And he will put a yoke of iron on your neck until he has destroyed you. (Deuteronomy 28:47-48)**

When the people of Israel wanted a king like the world, God's heart wanted David to be king of Israel. David became Israel's second king. It was a difficult journey to the throne, yet God knew that David would act according to His will.

> **And when he had removed him [Saul], he raised up David to be their king, of whom he testified and said, 'I have found in David the son of Jesse a man after my heart, who will do all my will.' (Acts 13:22)**

David made some serious mistakes during his time as king. He encountered some terrifying and heartbreaking situations and cried out to the Lord, but he never grumbled against the Lord. He always acknowledged God's goodness and justice. He never accused God of being unfair or complained about His instruction. He always deferred his situations, his sin, his feelings, and his fear to the Lord's just judgment. He trusted God completely.

David stayed humble. He showed mercy and love to his enemies. He loved the Lord with every bit of his heart and worshipped Him with all he had in him. David was never afraid of the outcome. He was willing to lay down his crown and step away from the throne, knowing if it was God's will, He would bring him back.

> **For David had done what was right in the eyes of the LORD and had not turned aside from anything the LORD commanded all the days of his life, except in the matter of Uriah the Hittite. (1 Kings 15:5 BSB)**

In the 23rd Psalm, David writes, "The Lord is my shepherd, **<u>I shall not want</u>**". He trusted God to provide, but also treated this as a command. He shall not – will not – want. He **shall not want more** than God gives Him. He **shall not want his own will** to be done. He **shall not want his way**. He **shall be satisfied** with what the Lord has given. Having the Lord with him was enough for him. He feared the Lord and knew He was sovereign. He accepted that God gives and takes away, and He is right and just for doing so.

*David knew not to complain or question God's decisions, even when it was unpleasant for him. He also knew He could take his complaints before the Lord, but that He must do it humbly, knowing that God's will was perfect.*

**Do all things without grumbling or questioning, that you may be blameless and innocent, children of God without blemish in the midst of a crooked and twisted generation, among whom you shine as lights in the world, Philippians 2:14-15**

*David knew Israel's tendencies to run away from God to serve idols. As king, he would not let that happen, but Israel was not much different than we are today. When they couldn't get what they wanted from God's ways, they tried to get it elsewhere.*

---

**"So many today are not content with our perfect God. They think they can tweak Him and His commands to fit their mold, their agenda, and their ways. From the outside many appear to be living the so-called Christian life, but something is not quite right. It doesn't quite click because instead of leading others away from sin, there tends to be a leading towards sin, whether in idolatry or other sin.**

**There must be an opening of our eyes to see all that the Lord has given us, <u>to be content</u>, to obey His commands, and to see the Lord correctly that His ways are perfect and true, as well as see ourselves rightly.**

**Throughout the Old Testament I have noticed God repeating 'Follow my commands and statutes and walk in my ways'; it's a command He gives. There is no veering to the right or the left and doing it slightly our way, why? Because our way leads to death; His way leads to life! It saddens me to see so many deceived, as the saying goes, 'We can have our cake and eat it too' type Christians out there."**

*−Alysha Allen (Used with permission)*

---

*Our God is a god of wrath against the wicked, but He is also the God of grace that made a way, and guides us along that way, to his righteousness. He is the God who has done for us what we could not do for ourselves – save us from our wicked nature. Yes, this is the God who gave you your life at the cost of His own son's life. The God who provides all your needs, protects you, and comforts you in your trials. Why wouldn't He be offended by your complaints?*

**It was also about these that Enoch, the seventh from Adam, prophesied, saying, "Behold, the Lord comes with ten thousands of his holy ones, to execute judgment on all and to convict all the ungodly of all their deeds of ungodliness that they have committed in such an ungodly way, and of all the harsh things that ungodly sinners have spoken against him." <u>These are grumblers, malcontents, following their own sinful desires; they are loud-mouthed boasters, showing favoritism to gain advantage.</u> (Jude 1:14-16)**

God wants cheerful givers, with hearts of gratitude. He abhors grumbling. When we complain about our lives, our situations, others, or ourselves, we are complaining against God.

> **And Moses said, "When the Lord gives you in the evening meat to eat and in the morning bread to the full, because the Lord has heard your grumbling that you grumble against him—what are we? Your grumbling is not against us but against the Lord." (Exodus 16:8)**

When you declared that God was Lord (or master) of your life, you gave up your right to be lord. When you told Him, "You will be my God!", that means that you can no longer be your own god. What right do you have to complain when your life belongs to Him?

- **For the sake of Christ, then, I am content with weaknesses, insults, hardships, persecutions, and calamities. For when I am weak, then I am strong. (2 Corinthians 12:10)**

- **Not that I am speaking of being in need, for I have learned in whatever situation I am to be content. I know how to be brought low, and I know how to abound. In any and every circumstance, I have learned the secret of facing plenty and hunger, abundance and need. (Philippians 4:11-12)**

- **Keep your life free from love of money, and be content with what you have, for he has said, "I will never leave you nor forsake you." (Hebrews 13:5)**

- **Now there is great gain in godliness with contentment, for we brought nothing into the world, and we cannot take anything out of the world. But if we have food and clothing, with these we will be content. (1 Timothy 6:6-8)**

- **And he said to them, "Take care, and be on your guard against all covetousness, for one's life does not consist in the abundance of his possessions." (Luke 12:15)**

- **Now there is great gain in godliness with contentment. (1 Timothy 6:6)**

- **"Blessed are those who hunger and thirst for righteousness, for they shall be satisfied. (Matthew 5:6)**

- **The fear of the Lord leads to life, and whoever has it rests satisfied; he will not be visited by harm. (Proverbs 19:23)**

- **Better is a handful of quietness than two hands full of toil and a striving after wind. (Ecclesiastes 4:6)**

## I Shall Not Want

*(This page is printable and sharable)*
The Hope of Ruth Ministries ©2021 Heather Phipps

# Fear of God and Man

## To Fear, or Not to Fear?

The Lord commands at least 82 times in scripture that we should "fear the Lord" or have a "fear of the Lord". It is in the purpose behind the first commandment he gives to the people in Deuteronomy. In Isaiah 11, the fear of the Lord is one of the Spirits of God.

*That you may <u>fear the Lord your God</u>, you and your son and your son's son, by keeping all his statutes and his commandments, which I command you, all the days of your life, and that your days may be long.... You shall love the Lord your God with all your heart and with all your soul and with all your might. And these words that I command you today shall be on your heart." (Deuteronomy 6:2, 5-6)*

*There shall come forth a shoot from the stump of Jesse, and a branch from his roots shall bear fruit. And the Spirit of the Lord shall rest upon him, the Spirit of wisdom and understanding, the Spirit of counsel and might, the Spirit of knowledge <u>and the fear of the Lord</u>. And his delight shall be in the fear of the Lord. He shall not judge by what his eyes see, or decide disputes by what his ears hear.*
*(Isaiah 11:1-3)*

So, does God really want us to be terrified of him? Scripture often tells us not to be afraid. This can be confusing for believers. What exactly is the fear of the Lord?

To those in the world, the fear of the Lord should be terrifying.

*And the fear of the Lord fell upon all the kingdoms of the lands that were around Judah, and they made no war against Jehoshaphat. (2 Chronicles 17:10)*

For us, however, it is knowing the **fear of not being in right standing with the Lord**. It is **knowing the might and power and righteousness of our God**. It is **standing in awe** of who He is and what He does. It is **knowing He gives and takes away; He is a just and righteous judge**. It is **accepting His discipline** and **hating sin**. It is **trusting the Lord's sovereignty** in every situation in our lives. It is **believing** His word is true, and that He will do what He says He will do. **It is humility**, keeping God in His rightful place as God, and us in our rightful place as His servants. **Knowing we are the clay – not the Potter**. It is **loving Him more than self**, putting **Him first** in our lives. It is **obedience** and **wisdom**.

*"See now that I, even I, am he, and there is no god beside me; I kill and I make alive; I wound and I heal; and there is none that can deliver out of my hand." (Deuteronomy 30:39)*

*You will say to me then, "Why does he still find fault? For who can resist his will?" But who are you, O man, to answer back to God? Will what is molded say to its molder, "Why have you made me like this?" Has the potter no right over the clay, to make out of the same lump one vessel for honorable use and another for dishonorable use? What if God, desiring to show his wrath and to make known his power, has endured with much patience vessels of wrath prepared for destruction, in order to make known the riches of his glory for vessels of mercy, which he has prepared beforehand for glory. (Romans 9:19- 23)*

*Why do you serve the Lord? Do you serve from an obligation? Do you serve to avoid hell? Or do you serve Him because you fear him and love him and know He alone is worthy of your love?*

**"Hear, O Israel: The Lord our God, the Lord is one. You shall love the Lord your God with all your heart and with all your soul and with all your might. And these words that I command you today shall be on your heart. You shall teach them diligently to your children, and shall talk of them when you sit in your house, and when you walk by the way, and when you lie down, and when you rise. (Deuteronomy 6:4-7)**

## Fear the Lord – Not Man

Why fear the opinions of people? Why are you worried about impressing your coworkers, boss, neighbors, or friends? Do you fear their rejection if your thoughts, words, or actions offend them? They have no power over your soul. **Trying to please others often puts you at odds with God.** It is better to fear the Lord and His thoughts about you than any man's opinions. It is better to worry about offending God than offending people. Better to risk the rejection of man than rejection from the Lord!

**And do not fear those who kill the body but cannot kill the soul. Rather fear him who can destroy both soul and body in hell. (Matthew 10:28)**

**I tell you, my friends, do not fear those who kill the body, and after that have nothing more that they can do. But I will warn you whom to fear: fear him who, after he has killed, has authority to cast into hell. Yes, I tell you, fear him! (Luke 12:4-5)**

**For am I now seeking the approval of man, or of God? Or am I trying to please man? If I were still trying to please man, I would not be a servant of Christ. (Galatians 1:10)**

**The fear of man lays a snare, but whoever trusts in the Lord is safe. (Proverbs 29:25)**

**Saul said to Samuel, "I have sinned, for I have transgressed the commandment of the Lord and your words, because I feared the people and obeyed their voice. (1 Samuel 15:24)**

**So we can confidently say, "The Lord is my helper; I will not fear; what can man do to me?" (Hebrews 13:6)**

**The Lord is on my side; I will not fear. What can man do to me? (Psalm 118:6)**

**When I am afraid, I put my trust in you. In God, whose word I praise, in God I trust; I shall not be afraid. What can flesh do to me? (Psalm 56:3-4)**

**But even if you should suffer for righteousness' sake, you will be blessed. Have no fear of them, nor be troubled. (1 Peter 3:14)**

**"I, I am he who comforts you; who are you that you are afraid of man who dies, of the son of man who is made like grass". (Isaiah 51:12)**

*The Fear of the Lord Defined*

*The Fear of the Lord is:*

- *A requirement – **(Deuteronomy 10:12)***
  **And now, Israel, what does the Lord your God require of you, but to fear the Lord your God, to walk in all his ways, to love him, to serve the Lord your God with all your heart and with all your soul.**

- *Hatred of evil – **(Proverbs 8:13)***
  **The fear of the Lord is hatred of evil. Pride and arrogance and the way of evil and perverted speech I hate.**

- *Respecting God's authority (obedience) – **(Genesis 22:12)***
  **He said, "Do not lay your hand on the boy or do anything to him, for now I know that you fear God, seeing you have not withheld your son, your only son, from me."**

- *Wisdom – **(Psalm 111:10)***
  **The fear of the Lord is the beginning of wisdom; all those who practice it have a good understanding. His praise endures forever!**

- *Awe – **(Psalm 33:8)***
  **Let all the earth fear the Lord; let all the inhabitants of the world stand in awe of him!**

- *Reverent fear – **(Hebrews 11:7)***
  **By faith Noah, being warned by God concerning events as yet unseen, in reverent fear constructed an ark for the saving of his household. By this he condemned the world and became an heir of the righteousness that comes by faith.**

- *Terror on His enemies – **(2 Chronicles 17:10)***
  **And the fear of the Lord fell upon all the kingdoms of the lands that were around Judah, and they made no war against Jehoshaphat.**

- *Fountain of Life – **(Proverbs 14:27)***
  **The fear of the Lord is a fountain of life, that one may turn away from the snares of death.**

- *Strong Confidence – **(Proverbs 14:26)***
  **In the fear of the Lord one has strong confidence, and his children will have a refuge.**

- *Complete Holiness – **(2 Corinthians 7:1)***
  **Since we have these promises, beloved, let us cleanse ourselves from every defilement of body and spirit, bringing holiness to completion in the fear of God.**

- *Trust – **(Psalm 115:11)***
  **You who fear the Lord, trust in the Lord! He is their help and their shield.**

- *Rewarded with Blessings, Friendship of the Lord, No lack, and God's compassion.*
  **(Psalm 112:1)  Blessed is the man who fears the Lord, who greatly delights in his commandments!**
  **(Psalm 25:14)  The friendship of the Lord is for those who fear him**
  **(Psalm 34:9)  Those who fear him have no lack!**
  **(Psalm 103:13) The Lord shows compassion to those who fear him.**
  **(Proverbs 22:4) The reward for humility and fear of the Lord is riches and honor and life.**

# The Self-god

*For rebellion is as the sin of witchcraft, and stubbornness is as iniquity and idolatry.*
*(1 Samuel 15:23 BSB)*

As a Christian, you probably believe you are far from the sin of idolatry and witchcraft. Yet, if you are like most people, you have stubborn and rebellious moments. The verse above may have you wondering, "What exactly is idolatry and witchcraft?

Witchcraft involves a manipulation of circumstances powered by the demonic. It is often blatant occultic practices – most likely things you don't do. Yet, **at the heart** of witchcraft is the desire to know the future and control events that are not ours to control, abilities that belong only to the Lord. It is the desire to be in control that causes rebellion. Can you see the similarity to witchcraft? The Lord looks at the heart. **A rebellious heart is the same condition of the heart willing to perform witchcraft.**

In rebellion, we attempt to make situations line up with our desires instead of seeking the Lord's will. We attempt to control how our life will go, instead of accepting the Lord's will for our life. We try to manipulate circumstances to our benefit and our ways, instead of relying on God's ways. We want to fast-track the path we are on or define our destiny as we want it. We may even attempt to control or manipulate another person's will to line up with our will. This is the core purpose of witchcraft.

Do you grumble and complain? How are you unsatisfied with life? What do you try to control? The answers to these questions can help you spot rebellion in your heart.

Idolatry is not the same as witchcraft. I searched scripture to define idolatry and found Colossians 3:5, but I noticed some differences within the translations.

### Colossians 3:5

*Therefore put to death your members which are on the earth: fornication, uncleanness, passion, evil desire, and covetousness, which is idolatry. (New King James Version)*

*Put to death therefore what is earthly in you: sexual immorality, impurity, passion, evil desire, and covetousness, which is idolatry. (English Standard Version)*

*You must put to death, then, the earthly desires at work in you, such as sexual immorality, indecency, lust, evil passions, and greed (for greed is a form of idolatry). (Good News Translation)*

*So put to death the sinful, earthly things lurking within you. Have nothing to do with sexual immorality, impurity, lust, and evil desires. Don't be greedy, for a greedy person is an idolater, worshiping the things of this world. (New Living Translation)*

The first two translations appear to give a list of things that are idolatry, but the last two state it is only greed. **To find out if all these works of the flesh were idolatry or if it was just greed, I looked up how the phrase "which is idolatry" was translated from the Greek.**

The word used for "which" was hétis (hay-tis); it can mean whoever, anyone, or someone of such a nature, but this particular usage of the word serves to give a reason. It is equivalent to saying, "seeing that he did this" or "inasmuch as he did that".

The word used for "idolatry" is eidólolatria (i-do-lol-at-ri'-ah). This is fairly straight forward. The definition is image worship; the service (worship) of an image (an idol).

So, Colossians 3:5 could be read to say:

> Put to death therefore what is earthly in you: sexual immorality, impurity, passion, evil desire, and covetousness, **seeing that you are worshipping an image**

It could also just as accurately be translated:

> Put to death therefore what is earthly in you: sexual immorality, impurity, passion, evil desire, and covetousness, **inasmuch as you are in the service of an idol.**

Let's read 1 Samuel 15:23 again.

**"For rebellion is as the sin of witchcraft, and stubbornness is as iniquity and idolatry."**

**Witchcraft is a response to idolatry just as rebellion is an action that results from stubbornness.** God is sovereign. He is in control, but we want control. We want to change situations to benefit our will. We want our will to be done on earth. Our stubbornness is equated to idolatry. It is the heart condition that promotes the rebellion. Our acts of rebellion are like performing witchcraft. Being stubborn against the ways of God is the worship of a false god or idol. **So, rebellion is an <u>act of worship</u> to a false god, and the god is you.** When you seek knowledge, power, or spirituality apart from God, it is idolatry, and puts you in rebellion to God's sovereignty.

Satan is full of pride and hate. He hates you because you have a resemblance of God. If he can divert your heart away from worshipping the true God and entice you with the idea of self-power, control, self-realization, or spiritual enlightenment apart from submission to the authority of the Lord Almighty, He destroys the image of God in you eternally.

## The Anti-God Battle

Satan excels in counterfeiting what God does. Do you remember the magicians, who by demonic power, created counterfeits of the miracles Moses performed before Pharaoh? Today, he continues to counterfeit the authentic.

Mankind was created in a divine nature, not as gods, but without sin, like God. In the Garden of Eden, mankind walked with God, and He gave mankind all authority and dominion of the earth, except one thing. He told Adam the one thing he may not do was to eat of the tree of the knowledge of good and evil. The one thing God said mankind could not do was to decide for himself what was good or evil. Once we decided for ourselves what was good and bad, we also decided what was right and wrong, thus creating our own morality apart from the Lord.

*We continue in this same sin today. We decide for ourselves what is right and wrong, and we become the arbiters of justice. We redefine what God calls good and corrupt it – we create a counterfeit, in the same way Satan creates counterfeits.*

*Satan wanted to rule; he wanted God's throne. He wanted to show himself mightier than God.* **In the garden, Satan created the beginning of an army of servants who would go fourth counterfeiting God's good design and corrupting His plan, His will, and His word for generations.**

*So, now we see why the Lord is right and just to destroy the wicked. Why He is right to demand no other God before Him, and that He is sovereign. His jealousy is righteous. His ways are good because even before he created the opportunity to choose wrong, he made the escape route. He had the plan of salvation in place before the foundations of the world were laid.*

> **For if these qualities are yours and are increasing, they keep you from being ineffective or unfruitful in the knowledge of our Lord Jesus Christ. <u>For whoever lacks these qualities is so nearsighted that he is blind, having forgotten that he was cleansed from his former sins.</u>**
> **(2 Peter 1-8-9)**

*When you choose the ways of your flesh – or your own understanding, seeking knowledge or control outside of God – you become blind, near-sighted – only looking at the situation right in front of you, or dissecting the details of a situation into oblivion trying to make sense of or control something that is not yours to know or control. You forget who you are and who you belong to. God is your master, your lord. He owns you. He paid a hefty price, the life of His Son, for you. And He is Sovereign.*

## The Anti-Christ Flesh

*If worshipping your flesh is idolatry and idolatry is the worship of an image, what image are you worshipping when you indulge your flesh? You might say your own image, you are worshiping self. We are made in the image of God – yet these things are contrary to God, or anti-God. Therefore, the image we are worshipping is an anti-god image.*

> **For the mind that is set on the flesh is hostile to God,**
> **for it does not submit to God's law; indeed, it cannot. (Romans 8:7)**

> **For the desires of the flesh are against the Spirit, and the desires of the Spirit are against the flesh, for these are opposed to each other, to keep you from doing the things you want to do. (Galatians 5:17)**

**Who owns you?** *You are either owned by your sin and the world, which falls under the dominion of the enemy, or you are owned by God. The world hates you. It is out for itself. Your sin deceives you. It cares only about the moment and cannot perceive what is truly good. The only power your sin has is to destroy and decay. It rots your soul and* kills you. God on the other hand, loves you. He plans a future for you, an eternal future. He gives you hope, peace and joy. He wants good for you and is generous and selfless.

*Do you not know that if you present yourselves to anyone as obedient slaves, you are slaves of the one whom you obey, either of sin, which leads to death, or of obedience, which leads to righteousness? (Romans 6:16)*

What are the things of the flesh that we worship?

*"Now the works of the flesh are evident: sexual immorality, impurity, sensuality, idolatry, sorcery, enmity, strife, jealousy, fits of anger, rivalries, dissensions, divisions, envy, drunkenness, orgies, and things like these. I warn you, as I warned you before, that those who do such things will not inherit the kingdom of God." (Galatians 5:19-21)*

If you are causing dissention and divisions, gossip, attention seeking, could it be that power and acceptance are your gods? Is sex your god? Rivalries and fits of anger? Could success and money be your gods? What about your phone? Social media? Entertainment? Your job or your status? Perhaps it is your friends or your family that are your god? Anything at all that you **put above** God, **value more** than God, **take time away from God** to do, or that you would **rebel against God** to do, that is your idol.

We are to love God with **all** our heart, mind, and soul. When we are acting in our flesh, being disobedient to God, we are against him. **If we are not for Him, we are against Him.** We are not loving God; we are loving the world and become an enemy of God. **We are not worshipping Christ. We are worshipping the anti-Christ**.

I am **not** talking about worshipping the man called the Anti-christ who is coming to wreak havoc on this world. I am speaking about you. Every idol mentioned above glorifies you. The one being worshipped is your own self above God.

*Do not love the world or anything in the world. If anyone loves the world, the love of the Father is not in him.  For all that is in the world—the desires of the flesh, the desires of the eyes, and the pride of life—is not from the Father but from the world. The world is passing away, along with its desires; but whoever does the will of God remains forever.  Children, it is the last hour; and just as you have heard that the antichrist is coming, so now many antichrists have appeared. This is how we know it is the last hour.* <u>*They went out from us, but they did not belong to us. For if they had belonged to us, they would have remained with us.*</u> *But their departure made it clear that none of them belonged to us. (1 John 2 15-19)*

This scripture speaks of people in the church being exposed and separated in the last hour, which we are certainly in. Many people will come with a form of godliness and an outward appearance of Christ, but inwardly deny the power of the true God and are ravenous wolves. People worshipping self and their flesh more than the Lord will be separated from the fold because their hearts are not genuinely for the Lord. They have not circumcised the flesh of their heart.  **Is this you?**

# The Self-lover

## God Respects Himself

God knows He is worthy of respect, there is none equal to him, none who compares to Him. He sees Himself as worthy, and He demands the respect he deserves. God loves Himself, and commands us to love Him also, as well as ourselves and others. You cannot love your neighbor as yourself if you do not love yourself.

## Love Your Neighbor as Yourself

**"Loving others as yourself" shows us how we are to treat ourselves as much as it shows us how to treat others.** You may know it is wrong to harm another person with your words, yet you harm yourself with your own thoughts and words. You may cover over another person's wrongs in love yet beat yourself up for your own wrongs. You may forgive another and not forgive yourself. Or vice-versa. You may ignore your faults and blame others. You may gossip about others to build your own confidence and cover your own flaws. Neither are love. Thus, loving others as yourself is a command to love both other people and you.

*Don't take vengeance on or bear a grudge against any of your people; rather, love your neighbor as yourself; I am Adonai. (Leviticus 19:18)*

*Rather, treat the foreigner staying with you like the native-born among you — you are to love him as yourself, for you were foreigners in the land of Egypt; I am Adonai your God. (Leviticus 19:34)*

*'And you shall love the Lord your God with all your heart and with all your soul and with all your mind and with all your strength.' The second is this: 'You shall love your neighbor as yourself.' There is no other commandment greater than these. (Mark 12:30-31)*

*And he said to him, "You shall love the Lord your God with all your heart and with all your soul and with all your mind. This is the great and first commandment. And a second is like it: You shall love your neighbor as yourself. (Matthew 22:37-39)*

*Honor your father and mother, and, You shall love your neighbor as yourself. (Matthew 19:19)*

*And he answered, "You shall love the Lord your God with all your heart and with all your soul and with all your strength and with all your mind, and your neighbor as yourself." (Luke 10:27)*

*If you really fulfill the royal law according to the Scripture, "You shall love your neighbor as yourself," you are doing well. (James 2:8)*

*For the whole law is fulfilled in one word: "You shall love your neighbor as yourself." (Galatians 5:14)*

*For the commandments, "Don't commit adultery," "Don't murder," "Don't steal," "Don't covet," and any others are summed up in this one rule: "Love your neighbor as yourself." (Romans 13:9)*

*Loving Yourself vs Being a Lover of Self*

There is a distinction between loving yourself and being lovers of self.

**But understand this, that in the last days there will come times of difficulty. For people will be lovers of self, lovers of money, proud, arrogant, abusive, disobedient to their parents, ungrateful, unholy, heartless, unappeasable, slanderous, without self-control, brutal, not loving good, treacherous, reckless, swollen with conceit, lovers of pleasure rather than lovers of God, having the appearance of godliness, but denying its power. Avoid such people. (2 Timothy 3:1-5)**

God condemns being a lover of self. The difference between loving yourself and being a lover of self is how you treat others and the value you place on your eternal soul.

**Whoever gets sense loves his own soul; he who keeps understanding will discover good. (Proverbs 19:8)**

What are you loving when you love your soul? You love the new creation you are becoming in Christ. You love your eternal soul, your eternal existence with God. You place eternity as having a higher value than this life. Understanding this you will "discover good". You will keep the Lord's commands because you love your soul enough to protect it from eternal consequences.

**If you are loving yourself, you respect yourself and want others to treat you well.** You, therefore, can treat other people the way you would like to be treated. When you love yourself, you are not in competition with others. You can give them honor, because you know that you are honorable and do not need the recognition. Therefore, you can show others a high regard, esteem them, build them up, without taking credit for yourself.

**"So whatever you wish that others would do to you, do also to them, for this is the Law and the Prophets. (Matthew 7:12)**

**Do nothing from selfish ambition or conceit, but in humility count others more significant than yourselves. (Philippians 2:3)**

**A lover of self, however, is one with selfish love.** A love of self that seeks the approval of man above all else. It looks after its own ego and pride and does not humble itself before God. Such a person does not love his eternal soul, rather he loves his sinful flesh. He does not desire the will of God, but his own will to be done. His ambitions are selfish. His motives seek to please and glorify himself.

*God Leads by Example*

The Lord tells us to love others as we love ourselves. He leads by example. He loves us as himself laying down his own life for ours. He respects us through his compassion and mercy, and He expects us to return that respect to him through our obedience. He respects us in our weakness and expects us to respect his authority.

# Valuable or Worthy

*I once heard an illustration about a $1 bill. You can crumple up, stomp on, spit on, and totally mistreat a $1 bill, but when you pick it back up, it still retains the value of one dollar. The thought was that no matter what life does to you, it doesn't take away your value. The question I debated was, "Is this true?" Can the enemy actually shred the $1 bill, (you) to a point where it is beyond repair? Can he shred your heart to a point that you lose your value.*

***Value is potential worth.*** *If you think about selling a car you may check its book value. Exchanging the car has the potential to redeem a certain amount of treasure. But it's true worth is only what the purchaser is willing to pay for it.*

*Your car may have a book **value** of $1000 but if you can only find someone willing to give you $300 for it, it is really only **worth** $300 to you, right. On the other hand, if you **believe** the car has a **value** of $4000, but if the **actual sale price** at auction is $10,000, you **underestimated its worth.** You were unable to see the value in what you had.*

*Are you valuable? Yes, you are! Every person from birth is valuable. God made each person unique and there will never be another like them in personality and character. No one else will think just like them or have the same ideas, visions, or heart. You have value because there will never be another like you with your unique traits, calling, and potential. God created you for a specific purpose which gives your life value. **Yet, the fact a person exists does not give them worth.***

## What determines your worth?

***The worth of something is determined by the one who redeems its value.*** *The one who redeemed the car for $10,000 instead of $4000, gave the car its worth. Likewise, **it is who redeems a person who gives them worth**.*

*If a person tries to get their worth from the "world", they are trying to get their worth from the principalities who rule this fallen world. For the believer to seek their worth in the world, is to desire their enemy to value them, and that's not going to happen.*

**Do not be surprised, brothers and sisters, that the world hates you. (1 John 3:13)**

*To attempt to earn your value in the world, means you must seek its approval. To become friends with the world makes you God's enemy.*

***You adulterous people! Do you not know that friendship with the world is enmity with God? Therefore whoever wishes to be a friend of the world makes himself an enemy of God. (James 4:4)***

*There is no worth in our sin nature except what we give to ourselves. You will hear the world speak about "self-esteem". Why do you need to esteem yourself? Because no one in this world will esteem you, for you.*

*Worldly people will praise good deeds. So, your worth becomes entangled in your ability to be good. What happens when you screw up? They praise helpfulness and philanthropy. Your worth depends upon your ability to help others. What happens when you are the one in need? They admire success, power, and money. What happens when you fail, have financial setbacks, or someone more powerful comes along? Where does your worth go?* **Your worth is at the mercy of another person's opinion.**

*What happens in a world of people striving to find belonging, acceptance, and worth – anything to prove they are somehow important? You find a world full of hate. People shouting, rioting, looting, gossiping, backbiting, lying, scheming and belittling others. People who need to be seen, to matter, and have their voices heard at any cost.*

*Seeking value in the world places a higher and higher expectation on you to always do something more, have something more, be something better – and a person will never reach the end. They will never be enough for the world. The world will* **never** *value them as they are, and their worthless pursuits will make them worthless.*

> **Thus says the LORD: "What wrong did your fathers find in me that they went far from me, and went after worthlessness, and became worthless? (Jeremiah 2:5)**

> **Now the sons of Eli were worthless men. They did not know the LORD. (1 Samuel 2:12)**

> **A worthless witness mocks at justice, and the mouth of the wicked devours iniquity. (Proverbs 19:28)**

> **Whoever loves father or mother more than me is not worthy of me, and whoever loves son or daughter more than me is not worthy of me. And whoever does not take his cross and follow me is not worthy of me. (Matthew 10:37-38)**

**God's word says you have worth if** *you follow Jesus, know the Lord, put nothing before Him, and follow His ways. He says you are worthless if you mock his justice, seek after worthless things or if you do not know Him.*

*So, the answer to the $1 bill riddle is this.*

**The government is the only one with the authority to shred currency,** and **they only do this when taking it out of circulation**. *At that point it has no worth. It can no longer be redeemed and loses all value. But* **it is illegal for anyone else to destroy** *or mutilate currency in a way that makes it worthless. The dollar bill has and retains the value it was created with as long as it is in existence.*

**God is your government**. *He created you and gave you your initial value, equal to every other human being. He is the authority of* **every person** *regardless of their choice to see it or not.* **He is the only One with the authority to redeem you or decommission you.** *Your worth is determined when God decides if you are righteous in Christ, or worthless chaff to be burned up in the fire. The enemy cannot redeem you. He does not have the authority to give you worth or take it away.*

The ONLY one who can determine your worth is the one who determines your fate.

# The God Worthy to Give Worth

Maybe you are like me. I used to think, "It isn't that I don't trust God, I don't trust myself", or "I know that God can do anything, I'm just not sure He can with me.", or "I know God saved me, but I am too messed up to be used by Him."

While this sounds humble and faithful on the surface, in God's eyes, it shows a lack of faith. And the day I realized this; it broke my heart. You see, if God is sovereign over my life, if He changes my heart, if He makes me able, if He equips me to serve Him, if He gives and prepares me for my purpose and calling, then it is not about me at all.

What I am saying, by these seemingly humble remarks, is that I don't trust God is good enough, powerful enough, sovereign enough, to break my will. God is not stronger than I am. God can't handle me; I am too much of a challenge for Him. I was saying that God is not worthy to judge me as righteous. That is a very twisted pride.

On the other hand, I could find worth in myself from people's praise of my abilities or accomplishments. I found my worth in the people I respect standing in front of me. I saw them worthy to give me worth. Why couldn't I see God this way?

> *I have come in my Father's name, and you do not receive me. If another comes in his own name, you will receive him. How can you believe, when you receive glory from one another and do not seek the glory that comes from the only God? (John 5:43-44)*

Let's assume that a person of importance, say a president or ruler, one that you had respect and admiration for, approached you and wanted your advice or counsel about an issue. He felt you had something to offer. He asks you to serve with him. You feel value and worth because he sees your value. You receive worth from him because you believe that he is someone worthy to give you worth.

If a street criminal asked for your advice, it is unlikely you would feel the same sense of worth. Why not? You may fear him, but you would not find him worthy of honor or respect or admiration. He is not worthy to give you worth.

Remember, God created us, and He gives us value from birth. We become worthy when we choose God. He is the one who determines if we are redeemed. When we choose His ways by faith, He takes our sin and calls us righteous. Our guilt is paid, and we do not carry shame. He redeemed us for the highest price, the cost of His own son's life. He makes us worthy. Therefore, it is the Lord who gives us both our value and our worth.

> *Our ability to know our worth in God is directly related to how worthy we feel God is to give us that worth and value.*

How can you accept worth from someone who, in your eyes, is not worthy to give such a judgment? **if you do not find God worthy, then getting your value from him will make you feel worthless and** you would still feel the need to be validated **by someone else.**

*Who do you need to validate you?*

*Can you see the God of the Bible as who He truly is? He is the God of complete righteousness, who orchestrates the most finite details of history. He is the God who uses each facet of creation, each person, and every situation as an instrument in His orchestra to create a symphonic masterpiece.*

*If the intricacies of creation and the created do not persuade you of the majesty and wisdom of our God, or the provision and acts of God in your own life do not persuade you, then certainly the unfolding of the mysteries in the Bible should leave you in utter awe!*

*The meaning behind every name in Biblical history, in the genealogy of Jesus, creates the story of the coming Messiah. A genealogy guarded with the lives and nation of Israel, so they could identify their Messiah, and yet just as the scriptures said, they didn't know Him. They were blind. Books written over centuries, by different authors, in a history more carefully preserved than any other history, tell a consistent story. Prophecy unfolded so perfectly and precisely hundreds and thousands of years after it was given. How does this happen without a divine all-knowing hand behind it? It cannot.*

*No counterfeit can do these things! See the God worthy to give you worth!*

*Those who lack a personal relationship with God, who do not have the Fear of the Lord and sit in awe of the majesty of who He is and what He can do, will not recognize the simple fact that He is the one who decides their fate. As such, he is the only one able to give them value, worth, and purpose. They will spend their lives seeking, and never find, and in the end be left with bitter disappointment and an eternal fate separated from God. They are burned up in the fire as worthless chaff because they refused the worth they would be so freely given, had they only accepted it.*

*If you still think, "It is not God who isn't worthy – its me.", are you really saying He is not worthy to make that judgment? Or are you afraid of the judgment he will make?*

*Remember*

- *God determines if you are worthy or worthless.*
  **"For behold, the day is coming, burning like a furnace; and all the arrogant and every evildoer will be chaff; and the day that is coming will set them ablaze," says the Lord of hosts, "so that it will leave them neither root nor branch."(Malachi 4:1)**

- *The deciding factor is determined only by your love for God and obedience to Him.*
  **And now, Israel, what does the Lord your God require of you, but to fear the Lord your God, to walk in all his ways, to love him, to serve the Lord your God with all your heart and with all your soul, (Deuteronomy 10:12)**

# Man-made Truth

Defining religion is controversial and therefore difficult. Perhaps it can be best defined as a person's beliefs, values, and practices based on the teachings of a spiritual leader. The world is always creating its own religions or "world-views". Even if the belief is atheism (that there is no God or higher power) you have a religion. Think about it. If your beliefs, values, and practices are based on the teaching that there is an absence of a spiritual being, this is still a spiritual belief. Not only does the world deny God, but it also redefines Him and His ways as it sees fit.

As a Christian, you are probably very aware that worship of false gods, witchcraft, and idolatry are sins that have a steep and eternal consequence from the Lord. There are many specific things described in scripture that fall into these categories The obvious ones include sacrificing your child in the fire, divination or sorcery, witchcraft, spells, consulting or being a medium or spiritualist, consulting the dead, or interpreting omens. These people create their own truth apart from the Lord. Anyone who does these things is detestable to Him. You may think all Christians are far removed from witchcraft and idolatry as described in the scriptures, but let's take a deeper look.

## Occultic Christians?

Christians are no less guilty of defining truth than the world. Some ways are easy to spot through scripture. Perhaps you know of Christians who talk about deceased loved ones as their guardian angels, or who worship angels. God created the angels. They serve Him and minister to us. They watch us with interest because we are created in the image of their creator! We are not, nor do we become angels. Angel worship is idol worship.

> **And to which of the angels has he ever said, "Sit at my right hand until I make your enemies a footstool for your feet"? Are they not all ministering spirits sent out to serve for the sake of those who are to inherit salvation? (Hebrews 1:13-14)**

> **It was revealed to them that they were serving not themselves but you, in the things that have now been announced to you through those who preached the good news to you by the Holy Spirit sent from heaven, things into which angels long to look.**
> **(1 Peter 1:12)**

Perhaps you have heard a Christian talk about seeing or speaking to the spirit of a dead relative. Desperate for answers and healing, some believe this is a gifting from God, but the Bible clearly teaches that the dead and living cannot communicate. This is like consulting a medium. These people are deceived and communicating with demons.

> **"And he said, 'No, father Abraham, but if someone goes to them from the dead, they will repent.' He said to him, 'If they do not hear Moses and the Prophets, neither will they be convinced if someone should rise from the dead.'" (Luke 16:30-31)**

*Unfortunately, Satan has also infiltrated God's church in more subtle ways. He may not fool you with a blatant deception. He often deceives with partial truth.*

*I often hear Christians talk about karma? Some churches even offer Yoga for health, discounting it as a spiritual ritual. Yoga was first used by Brahmans, Vedic priests, and Rishis, who are mystic seers. It internalized the idea of ritual sacrifice, teaching the sacrifice of the ego through self-knowledge and action (karma yoga) and wisdom (jnana yoga). Karma is the antithesis of God's grace and the foundations of a false religion.*

*Many Christians discount pagan and occultic things as just fun. They see no harm in playing with a Ouija board, discounting that they open a real gateway to communicate with the demonic. "It is just a game sold in kid's stores."*

*They may play video or role-playing games that have spiritualism built in. They may read books or watch videos, television, or movies with vampires, demons, occult activity, or lude behavior. They may listen to music with lyrics that counter God's word, believing it is okay because they "know the truth" and they don't believe in these things.*

*Have you ever had your palm read at a festival? Do you pay attention to your astrological sign or look at your horoscope? Do you interpret omens, or interpret a circumstance to influence your actions? Do you rely on lucky numbers or keep good luck charms? These are occultic activities that replace prayer and discernment from God.*

### Is This Simply Overreacting to Harmless Fun?

*Satan uses the media to manipulate. There is little you can watch or listen to in entertainment that is not immersed with what God finds abhorrent. **Perhaps you don't see the problem with watching a television show** that has some lude behavior, vampires, demons, or occult activity. Maybe they are cute-ified, like a kids show with a puppy that finds a spell book and innocently reads an incantation, **but it has a moral story**! So, you allow your children to watch it.*

***What would the God, that you read about in scripture, think about Christian children being entertained by the occult simply because they are not practicing it?** Does that even make sense to you? This is like saying that it is okay to watch pornography because you are not physically engaged in it. **Not being physically engaged** in an act of immorality **does not mean that your heart is not engaged in it.***

> ***And he said, "What comes out of a person is what defiles him. For from within, out of the heart of man, come evil thoughts, sexual immorality, theft, murder, adultery, coveting, wickedness, deceit, sensuality, envy, slander, pride, foolishness. All these evil things come from within, and they defile a person." (Mark 7:20-23)***

*Satan is the prince of the air. He uses what we see and hear to sugar coat and delude the masses. He comes to devour like a roaring lion. **He wants that show to corrupt your child**. He wants that inuendo in that song to stick in your child's brain so when he reaches maturity it can have its full effect.*

*What we take into our minds becomes part of us, and the Lord warns us to **only** set our minds on what is right.*

**Finally, brothers, whatever is true, whatever is honorable, whatever is just, whatever is pure, whatever is lovely, whatever is commendable, if there is any excellence, if there is anything worthy of praise, think about these things. What you have learned and received and heard and seen in me—practice these things, and the God of peace will be with you. (Philippians 4:8-9)**

*Do not allow your mind to be filled with distractions of everything in the world around you through news or social media. God wants us to look at Him, not all the deception circling around us like vultures. Amazingly, you will not be uninformed about what you need to know. Remember He is sovereign, not us, so knowing all the spin changes nothing.*

### Redefining God's Truth in the Church

*There is much falsehood in the church today. It was a slow progression. Now it is hard to know what truth is. Who is the real God? Without the Holy Spirit helping you discern the scripture; you will be deceived. Test everything you read or hear in a sermon or music against the truth of God's word.*

**And they shall turn away their ears from the truth and shall be turned unto fables (2 Timothy 4:4).**

*In the 1950's, Science tried to replace God. Apologetics came about and tried to fight it, but by the 1960's the church faced moral issues and did not stand. They chose to be tolerant, but tolerating sin is not loving the sinner. They let sin go, and what started as ignoring sin, evolved in the church. Now many denominations of the church embrace sin as righteousness and God turns them over.*

*Both things continue as we walk forward in the original sin, defining for ourselves what is right and wrong and determining for ourselves what is truth. There is only one who defines truth. Only one who defines good and evil. And that is the LORD.*

*Today, the church has people embracing false, demonic, spirits masquerading as the Holy Spirit of God. People performing false miracles for a price, getting rich off the backs of desperate believers. Political social justice warriors have hitched a ride on the back of faith in an attempt to hijack a movement and gain power. Some churches embrace a greezy-feel-good-grace doctrine, refusing to preach any message that may offend, shouting legalism at the mention of morality, and leading people straight to hell.*

*A prosperity doctrine has infiltrated the church that drives people into depression or away from God because their success with Christ is dependent upon their ability to believe enough. The theology is one that implies you don't have what you want, not because of sin or because God has different plans, but because you are not believing enough. This leaves a person believing they are not good enough and a failure with God.*

*Legalistic doctrine completely dismisses the Spirit of God, dismisses women, dismisses the prophetic, or that any new thing could happen because it has already been done. They believe the word is all we have; God no longer speaks to his people. That is not truth!*

*A false, misleading, representation of our God and His word has people chasing signs and a goose-bump feeling. The Lord does confirm his thoughts and ways to us, but when the Lord gives you a sign, you should be able to back up what he is saying and how he is saying it, in the scripture. He will show you. God doesn't change, and the way He speaks to His people does not change either, yet our ability to hear him certainly has changed.*

**It is more important than ever to be solid in your word.**

- *Do not lean on prior understanding or teachings. Let the Lord teach you.*

- *Do not allow yourself to be spoon-fed the scripture from pastors or books.*

- *Seek the Holy Spirit as you read the Word of God for yourself!*

- *Learn the word. Read it all, and then read it again to study it deeper.*

- *Seek differences in translations and research the original language used.*

- *Learn about types and shadows in scripture.*

- *Allow the Holy Spirit to give understanding of parables.*

- *Take every verse in context with the entirety of scripture.*

- *Understand the original Jewish perspective of the passage you are reading.*

- *Use surveys of the Old and New Testament to learn about the culture and history of the time in which the scripture was written.*

# Regret

## What more can a man do about yesterday, than what He does, when the Lord makes everything new.

*Then I saw a new heaven and a new earth, for the first heaven and the first earth had passed away, and the sea was no more. And I saw the holy city, new Jerusalem, coming down out of heaven from God, prepared as a bride adorned for her husband. And I heard a loud voice from the throne saying, "Behold, the dwelling place of God is with man. He will dwell with them, and they will be his people, and God himself will be with them as their God. He will wipe away every tear from their eyes, and death shall be no more, neither shall there be mourning, nor crying, nor pain anymore, for the former things have passed away." And he who was seated on the throne said, "Behold, I am making all things new." Also he said, "Write this down, for these words are trustworthy and true." And he said to me, "It is done! I am the Alpha and the Omega, the beginning and the end. To the thirsty I will give from the spring of the water of life without payment. The one who conquers will have this heritage, and I will be his God and he will be my son. (Revelation 21:1-7)*

*"Behold, I am coming soon, bringing my recompense with me, to repay each one for what he has done. I am the Alpha and the Omega, the first and the last, the beginning and the end." Blessed are those who wash their robes, so that they may have the right to the tree of life and that they may enter the city by the gates. Outside are the dogs and sorcerers and the sexually immoral and murderers and idolaters, and everyone who loves and practices falsehood. "I, Jesus, have sent my angel to testify to you about these things for the churches. I am the root and the descendant of David, the bright morning star." The Spirit and the Bride say, "Come." And let the one who hears say, "Come." And let the one who is thirsty come; let the one who desires take the water of life without price. (Revelation 22:12-17)*

*And this is the will of him who sent me, that I should lose nothing of all that he has given me, but raise it up on the last day. For this is the will of my Father, that everyone who looks on the Son and believes in him should have eternal life, and I will raise him up on the last day." (John 6:39-40)*

Visit the website at:

*www.rebuiltrecovery.org*

for downloadable pages and
more helpful resources!

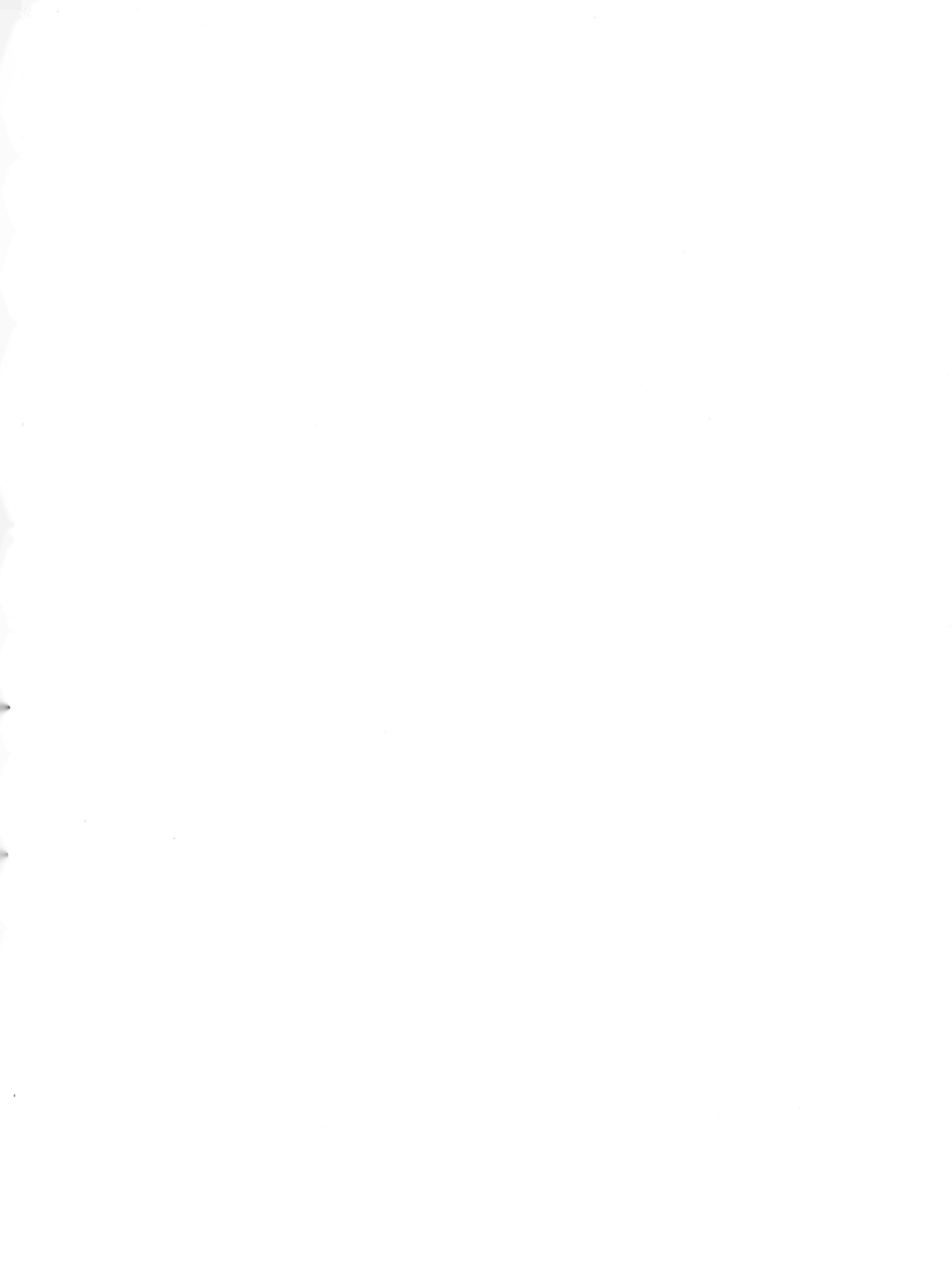